Scottish Nurses in the First World War

Scottish Nurses in the First World War

With the Scottish Nurses in Roumania
Yvonne Fitzroy

A History of the Scottish Women's
Hospitals
(Extract concerning service in the Balkans)
Eva Shaw McLaren

LEONAUR

Scottish Nurses in the First World War
With the Scottish Nurses in Roumania
by Yvonne Fitzroy
and
A History of the Scottish Women's Hospitals
(*Extract concerning service in the Balkans*)
by Eva Shaw McLaren

First published under the titles
With the Scottish Nurses in Roumania
and
A History of the Scottish Women's Hospitals
(*Extract concerning service in the Balkans*)

FIRST EDITION

Leonaur is an imprint
of Oakpast Ltd

ISBN: 978-1-78282-217-2 (hardcover)
ISBN: 978-1-78282-218-9 (softcover)

http://www.leonaur.com

Contents

With the Scottish Nurses in Roumania

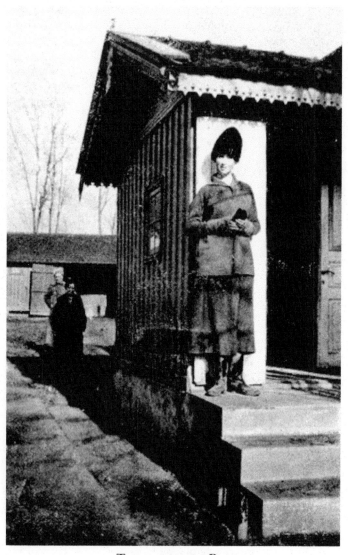

THE AUTHOR AT RENI

Contents

Foreword

It is to the memory of our beloved leader that the following pages are dedicated. I would do so in love and gratitude. Brief as was the time in which we were allowed to share in the great work of her life, the memory of its inspiration is, and will remain for ever, undying. Alongside the wider public loss, the full and noble public recognition, there stands in the shadow the unspoken sorrow of her Unit. The price has been paid, and paid as Dr. Inglis herself would have wished it on the high completion of a chapter in her work, but we stand bowed before the knowledge of how profound and how selfless was that surrender. Month after month her courage and her endurance never flagged. Daily and hourly, in the very agony of suffering and death, she gave her life by inches.

Sad and more difficult though the road must seem to us now, our privilege has been a proud one: to have served and worked with her, to have known the unfailing support of her strength and sympathy, and, best of all, to be permitted to preserve through life the memory and the stimulus of a supreme ideal.

Yvonne Fitzroy.

London, January, 1918.

CHAPTER 1

August—September

August 28th, 1916. Liverpool.

Just the wettest day you can imagine. My luggage consists of one kit-bag, one haversack, and a rug. Inside the rug I have concealed a fur-lined British warm—this against all rules and regulations.

The family and I arrived at Euston at 2. Mercifully one feels less oneself in this grey kit, and one's belongings have a super-military air which discourages the civilian emotions! Particularly the water-bottle; a real service one this, that seems to cry out for the battlefield and together with those lovely Red Cross labels "Russia," make the world enormous and all adventures possible. Nevertheless being seen off is not fun.

I travelled up with B. Here we are living very comfortably in the Station Hotel, and I, with supreme good luck, have got a room to myself. We reported to Miss H. our administrator, had dinner together, and went to bed.

It's exciting being alone—thoroughly and completely alone for the first time in one's life. It's quite different from being lonely. One is not that—yet. But to be alone in the sense of belonging thoroughly to oneself, not to have people around that expect anything of you or know anything about you. They've got to discover everything and so have you, because you don't the least know any more than they what you are going to do or to be like in this altogether new world. It's a dangerous, rocky kind of a feeling in a way, but it's stimulating, even now I wouldn't be missing it.

August 29th. Liverpool.

A comfortable night, and a very good breakfast. Most of the unit have assembled, some here and some at another hotel. We were free all the morning, so I roamed round the town, and bought a box of the very best Egyptian cigarettes with the remains of my English money! After luncheon the entire unit was photographed, and C. turned up, looking very smart in her khaki (Transport Section) uniform. The general public take a good deal of interest in us, and are divided in opinion as to whether we are a South Wales Regiment or merely a new form of girlguide.

We drove down to the docks about 4, and went on board the boat to get our passports. We are sailing on a ship captured from the Austrians in the Mediterranean, and we are told she is good, but she's not large, and is most exceedingly dirty.

B. and I share a cabin with another woman, who is certainly mad. We are lying close to the *Mauritania*. Got steam up about 10 p.m., and lay in the river all night.

August 31st. At Sea.
We weighed anchor about 8.30 p.m. A good speech from Dr. I., and life-belts were distributed and fitted on by a harassed steward, and then inspected by the captain. And so we have really and truly said goodbye, and have started.

September 1st. At Sea.
A heavy sea.

September 2nd. At Sea.
This morning we thought we really had met a submarine, but it turned out to be a whale!

I have missed everything today, including meals for obvious reasons.

September 3rd.
I awoke to a very calm sea, which was really comforting.

At 10.30 church parade. Dr. I. read very well. She gets more attractive every day. Tenacious, I should think, with a big brain.

At 4.30 Boat drill was sprung on us. Boat drill is a very wearing occupation. Just as you are happily curled up on deck there comes a piercing whistle. You rush to your cabin, you throw on your greatcoat, your life-belt and your water-bottle, and then rush back to your particular boat. Seventy-five other women are all rushing with you, and you emerge from the scrimmage looking, for all the world, like the famous poster for Michelin Tyres. One thing only—I trust they won't take to giving us these shocks at night.

16

We had a sing-song, and were out until 9.30. An infinitely big grey and silver sea. We have not seen land or sail for two days. At 10 p.m. we were heading East. They say, if the weather holds, we shall be at Archangel by Saturday.

September 4th. At Sea.

(*Extract from a letter.*)

We are feeling very content, for we had a lot of wireless news from England this morning.

It is a busy life that we lead—even now—at all moments when we are not *hors de combat.* This is the order of the day:

Breakfast, 8.30.
Roll Call and Inspection of Cabins, 9.30.
Military Drill, 10.30.
Swedish Drill, 11.
Luncheon, 12.30.
Sewing party. French and Russian Classes in the afternoon.
Tea, 4.
Serbian Class, 4.30.
Dinner, 6.30.
Bed any time.

This beautiful paper is the result of a few kind words to the purser. It might be cleaner, I allow, and the ship at the top is not the least like us. We are old, grubby, and grey—as I said before, Austrian.

I've only been laid up one day, and we started in beautiful weather.

September 6th.

We saw the *Aurora Borealis* last night. The Great White Bear and Pole Star lie directly ahead of us.

It sounds a poor description, but the searchlights at Hyde Park Corner give you the best idea of the Northern Lights. These might be huge and monumental ghosts of searchlights dead and gone, vague and wavering, that is if the Searchlight world is old enough to possess ghosts at all.

Most nights the Serbian soldiers sing, their own melancholy and very charming folk-songs.

This morning, just after breakfast, we entered the Arctic Circle.

I think you would laugh if you could see our Swedish Drill. All of us flat on our backs on the deck, waving our unaccustomed grey legs wildly in the air. Or the inebriated way in which we endeavour to form fours on the topsy-turvy deck. But as it is a sign of much health and strength to turn up at these functions most of us get there—pale but determined!

As far as I can make out the great majority of my fellow-workers are professionals—teachers very largely. B., the girl I travelled up with from Euston was at Girton, and as she survived the *Titanic* is, I feel, proof against all lesser disasters.

They are all pleasant.

September 7th.

The weather is as beautiful as ever. We are to touch at —— the day after tomorrow and, unless we are delayed, should reach Archangel on Sunday. Last night, there was quite an amusing dress-up concert. The Arctic Ocean can have rarely beheld a stranger company!

I have been gathering a good deal of information from the assistant matron. Our destination is very vague, as it depends on the movements of the troops. We are not to be under canvas during the winter, and may possibly stay at Odessa, but shan't go into winter quarters for a month or two yet. We are to form two hospitals.

I am learning Serb and sing the National Anthem in my bath.

September 8th. At Sea.

Floods of sunshine, the loveliest day we've had. Am appointed nursing orderly to Hospital A. under Dr. I. and am delighted. B. is in the same hospital as mess orderly.

September 9th. At Sea.

Reached at —— 3 a.m. One of our ships came out and told us to proceed straight to Archangel. We handed them over some mails for the English ships and left without putting in. Morning in the White Sea. A low brown shore not unlike a Scotch moor after the heather is over. A mail-bag was put up for our letters home. A wonderful pleasant sight.

We were given orders to take our rug-straps and haversacks only on the journey. Passed a whale and a lot of seals.

A wonderful evening, with a golden moon in a clear green sky, and a purple shore.

September 10th.

We reached Archangel after breakfast and lay just off the town. There is a curious flat shore, with short scrub, baby pine, and silver birch right down to the water's edge. The leaves are turning here and there. The houses are built of wood, with verandahs on the second and top storeys, and timber work is going on everywhere. The wharfs, too, are built of wood, and sometimes far out into the water on piles.

From the river the town looks just like a picture-book, with its towers of blue and gold, red and gold, and green and gold.

The river itself is full of shipping, and we anchored close to an English patrol yacht, looking beautifully the perfect lady amongst the grubby merchantmen and destroyers. Her commander came off on a launch and took Dr. I. ashore. The Excise and Custom House officials came aboard, and we were tugged to a dock opposite the new station about two miles up the river. How we cheered all the English boats, and how they cheered back!

For the rest of the day we were visited by officials of varying magnificence, and our surroundings are absorbing.

Great broad-bottomed barges pass, carrying a rough-looking kind of hay down stream, and sailing boats like Chinese *junks*. On shore there is a wonderful crowd, Russian and Mongolian, men, women and children, all in high boots, but after that following their own sweet wills in the fashion of their dress. Timber work is progressing in a leisurely fashion, and all by hand. The carts consist of a couple of planks and a log on two wheels, all driven by delightful children in huge fur caps. The soldiers are magnificent.

Dr. I. was back by tea-time. We are not to go to Petrograd, but to be sent straight through to Odessa. The Rumanian troops have had a defeat and the 1st Serbian Division has moved up to their assistance, the wounded are waiting for us, and there is no one else to help. So I am glad—but dreadfully disappointed that we shall miss our letters. Miss H. has telegraphed to have them sent on.

We were allowed on shore from 5.30 to 6.30, and had a good walk. Two Russian sentries with enormous bayonets held an animated conversation with us, and some French sailors gave us news from the Western Front. The crowds here are the most fascinating thing I have ever beheld, and the nights the most beautiful.

We entertained six nice washed naval officers to dinner, and had a concert afterwards. Colonel I., a Russian, at one time an opera singer, gave us *Tosca* and *Pagliacci*, and from these heights the programme drifted gracefully onward to a grand finale of "Tipperary."

September 11th.
A most unexpected 24 hours.
In the morning I went for a long walk over the docks with C. and

19

B. We saw a fascinating child in a red tunic and high red boots—height complete about 2 foot. The dock is strewn with munitions (so much so that we are not allowed to smoke on deck), guns and Armoured cars. After luncheon a launch came for the whole party and took us down to Archangel. We bought a vast store of chocolate and cigarettes, and Mrs. X. took us to see the Cathedral and Peter the Great's log hut. The wife of a big timber merchant, an Englishman, invited us all to tea in her garden. We made the most of this last really English meal and a gramophone!

On the way back in the launch the river looked beautiful, smoke coloured with the shipping, and the church towers silhouetted against a flaming heavily clouded sky.

To land we had to cross an open space above the water on two planks. B. and I were first off the boat. The planks were badly adjusted, they slipped off the wharf and tipped us both down a 20-foot drop into the water. I caught hold of a bar and B. of a ring which presented themselves just on the water-level, and after what seemed an eternity we were both hauled out.

Bed followed, with huge potations of brandy, hot-water bottles, a large dinner and the ministrations of two doctors, a matron, an assistant matron, two trained nurses and most of the ship's company. Our clothes are in a pitiable condition, not to mention all the good things we had bought in the town and with which our pockets were full. It is very, very sad!

September 12th. In the Train.

B. and I are very stiff, but none the worse. We got everything ready for leaving the ship, and took a short walk on the quay. Most of the others went to Archangel in the afternoon, but we were lazy, feeling too old. Roll Call at 6.30, and dinner at 7. We were then told to be ready and wait in the saloon. About 11 we lined up on the wharf. We marched to the train, carrying nearly all our worldly possessions and headed by the crew's patent band playing "Tipperary."

On the platform were two companies of Russian soldiers; they looked magnificent, and cheered as we came up. I found a sleeping-bunk along with F., T. and B., and then for 2½ hours while we waited for an engine the Russians entertained us. It was rather wonderful. Our boat all lit up as a background, the clearest of still, cold nights, and this great mass of shadowy figures shifting and moving as they sang and danced. Outside a fringe of peasants and Mongolians, just picturesque splashes of light and shadow. The dancing and singing were both a revelation and perfect. Sad songs they sing with a long slow rhythm.

It was such a contrast these big, impassive singing men and our own sailors who from beginning to end carried on a grotesque performance of their own in the background, of which "Tipperary," to an accompaniment of tin kettles, penny whistles, and a mouth-organ, was the most polished number. "Tipperary" I love, but oh—I could have killed that band!

Then everybody made speeches, and then we cheered everybody, and then everybody cheered us. Dr. I. and the officers were tossed This is a terrifying proceeding. The victim is thrust into a chair and hurled recklessly into the air up and down, while she clutches everything clutchable, tries to look appreciative and dignified, wonders if her hair will come down and hopes she won't be sea-sick, all at once. Dr. I. weathered the storm valiantly, and we all cheered to the echo.

Finally, between 1.30 and 2 a.m. we steamed slowly off. It was a very heartening welcome.

September 13th. In the Train.

A long day in the train and—Russia!

I don't quite know what we expected. Wolves, I suppose, and deep dark pine forests, with a Nihilist thrown in here and there as local colour. What we got was an attractive but unvarying country of birch and pine-wood. The timber is very small, here and there you come across a little wooden station, or a collection of toy wooden houses.

We travel very slowly and live on our own rations, which today consisted of:

Breakfast	bread and sardines.
Luncheon	bread and cheese.
Supper	bread and jam.

With our own supplies we did very well, The carriages are comfortable and quite fairly clean. There is no bedding of course, but we make ourselves comfortable at night in our own rugs and feel very superior with a whole train to ourselves. The cars are on trucks at the back and the equipment in waggons.

September 14th. In the Train.

We were woken up at 7 a.m. by an officer with the news that our couplings had broken in the night and that our carriage was marooned on the line.

Nothing surprises one in this country.

We flung on our clothes, and presently a horrible third-class compartment was sent to fetch us, and we were hitched on again. We spent the day getting bitten. Rations as usual, and I have acquired a filthy cold.

We reached Vologda at 11 p.m. Water is our great difficulty. There is little to drink, and none at all to wash in.

September 15th. In the Train.

We moved into a new sleeper carriage—very nice. Crossed the Volga, and reached Yaroslav about 2. A great big meal at the station— so good! The place was crowded. Jews, for the first time, Circassians and Cossacks. I rather expected everyone to be chanting the boat-song as a matter of course,—but they weren't!

September 16th. In the Train.

We were summoned early and told we should be in Moscow in ten minutes.

Rye bread and jam for breakfast. Rye bread I quite like; it's very sour, and you can't eat much of it, but it's good.

We continued to tour round and round outside Moscow until 3 in the afternoon. By that time everyone was terribly peevish and very hungry. Finally we reached the new station and were drawn up alongside a hospital train. Most of the station is used as a hospital, and the little Russian Sisters look delicious in their white *"religieuse"* caps. A Russian Red Cross potentate and his very pretty wife took us up to an hotel and gave us the most wonderful meal. Baths had to be sacrificed, but all the same we started for the *Kremlin* much refreshed. The trams set us down at the Saviour's Gate.

It's amazing. It's like walking into the *Arabian Nights*, into a great big fairy tale. A fairy palace over a fairy city and a fairy river.

Inside the little dim cathedrals there is an unending chant, long-haired priests are officiating, and soldiers, peasants, or Red Cross Sisters, looking like medieval nuns, wander to and fro. They are all in the picture; the place is never marred by the unromantic pew, and the soft-footed dimness is alive with colour. Ivan the Terrible and his two sons lie side by side in a tiny chapel opposite some wonderful fourteenth-century *ikons*. Outside, the evening light is a miracle. The city below seems all gold crosses and painted domes, the red brick outer walls of the citadel are glowing. It is beautiful this centre of Holy Russia—and mysterious—and—well, try travelling in a crowd for a

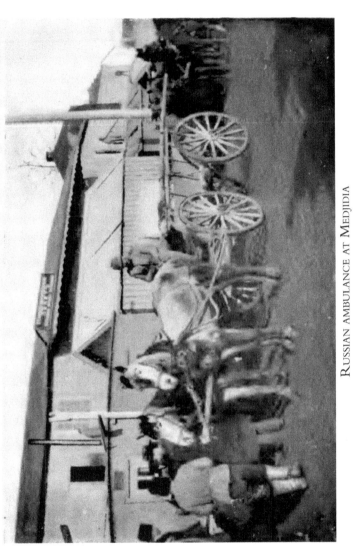

RUSSIAN AMBULANCE AT MEDJIDIA

week or two on ugly boats and trains, in ugly clothes, with a familiar and prosaic world behind you and, perhaps rather a terrible one to come, and then imagine what it feels like to be dropped suddenly for a short, short time into this strange Eastern City.

We Westerners seem, as it were, to have taken to ourselves all the credit of Christianity. We have torn it away from this East, and have said, "It is ours." In England particularly, with our talent far common-sense, we have robbed it of so much that is beautiful. As if we could got on without it! And why should religion not appeal to the imagination? Here, no doubt, it walks hand-in-hand with ignorance, but what hope is there in the future if we cannot look forward to a union between imagination and scientific knowledge?

The tomb of Ivan the Terrible, the Church of Ivan the Great, and the guns left by Napoleon tumbled us down the centuries to four great pieces of Austrian armament taken at Premysl just before the retreat.

We got back to the station in the dark, and in leisurely fashion we wandered over the line looking for our train. We discovered it eventually, and still more eventually started.

September 17th. In the Train.

Up early, a lovely morning, and I got quite a good wash. We had luncheon at a wayside station about 2. A lot of troop trains on the line and hospital trains full of wounded prisoners, Bulgars, Germans, and Austrians. At one stop we saw some Turks from Erzerum—poor devils. The peasants in their Sunday best came *en masse* to have a look at us. When we left they trotted cheering after the train. The railway seems to be the high road and resort of all who wish to see life in these parts.

Since Moscow the country is far more interesting and open. Women are working in the fields, on the railway, everywhere.

September 18th. In the Train.

Nothing very eventful to record. We had an excellent meal, and went shopping in a wayside village. The country very wide and open, and the timber bigger; maples turning the most gorgeous colours.

September 19th. In the Train.

We stopped at a most fascinating little wooden village for luncheon, though the filth was indescribable. It consisted of just one street, which was packed with open booths, peasants, beggars, and Jews.

These last are far the best-looking members of the community—great sad-looking men in gaberdines, as different as possible from the horrid type of little town Jew. The glimpses one gets into the conditions of the peasant's life are appalling.

We are even now afflicted with a horrible plague of flies.

Dr. I. had tea with the four of us. The other three all talked of their jobs before the War. I have always felt that the merely social existence must put one at a big disadvantage in the real world, but tonight I had to own up for the first time to the workers themselves. One does feel ashamed. But there is one comfort. It isn't that we others can't, it is that we haven't. We are beginning now, for which thank Heaven. We've got a long way to make up. In a life like this there are no frills, and we meet the workers on a level. We've got to do the job, and do it well—it's a great chance.

(Extract from a letter.)

It's very hot. Tea-parties are our great dissipation, and the food we alternately press on others and have pressed upon us is fearful and wonderful indeed. I am even having supper tonight with the ultra-exclusive transport!

September 20th. Tscherkassi.

The route *via* Kiev is too blocked, so ye have come this way and should arrive at Odessa Friday morning. Today we were let out—let out for a whole two hours—and we took a long walk across the *steppe* and into the town. We drove back to the station with much speed and considerable peril in a *droschki*. The driver's one object was, apparently, to avoid roads and drive as straight across country as circumstances would permit.

Oh for a bath!

September 21st. In the Train.

We were woken up with the tidings that we ought to be in Odessa by 7 o'clock tonight. I wonder if I shall sleep in a bed?

About 8 a.m. we crossed the Dnieper, and climbed up on to a magnificent open country—rather like the Downs, on an immense scale, burnt brown—the real Steppe.

We steamed into the station at Odessa about 7.30. On the platform were lined up the Serbian Staff and many glittering Russians. After a great interchange of *"politesse"* we in our turn were lined up and marched out. A humorous proceeding this, performed with complete gravity. At the door was a fleet of private *droschkis*. M., B. and I climbed into the foremost, and were whirled off by a grey Arab in black and silver harness. We raced the nearest party through the streets and won. It was wonderfully thrilling and wonderfully perilous. I didn't know horses could move like that.

We are the guests of the town, and they have housed us at a big sanatorium. Little one storey wooden houses in a nice garden and four or five of us lodged in each with—*real beds*. B., F., T., and I are again sharing a room, we are re-united to our kit-bags, and I have had a letter.

September 22nd. Odessa.

We suffered sad disillusion last night. Hardly had we done raving ecstatically about sheets and beds than a sinister thought struck each of us. We were too exhausted to move, but in the morning it was true—yes, the real beds had very real bugs in them as well! Bugs in such quantities indeed that it was quite useless to worry, and after ten days in the train even a buggy straw mattress is a preferable alternative to the floor.

This morning we retired across the road, where we were scrubbed in companies of five by extremely energetic old ladies. This is apparently the Russian custom. I don't mind washing in public when comparatively clean, but it requires a lot of courage when you are pale grey all over.

A Serbian soldier cleans our boots and a beautiful peasant girl— more Greek than any new thing I have ever seen—looks after us. She has bare feet and bare arms and a beautiful strong figure. Invariably she appears in a coarse *terra-cotta* coloured frock, with a white handkerchief tied round her head, and possesses a lovely face and neck a delicious person. Of course she *and* the Serb burst in at all moments, so dressing is never uneventful.

They give us meals in a big open-air dining-room, and the place is run by a colossal lady of Hebrew ancestry.

We spent rather an uninteresting and an extremely exhausting morning in the town. It is more Oriental, than Russian, the buildings are mostly modern, and there are Jews everywhere. Tomorrow we are going to *La Dame de Pique* at the opera.

Had my hair shampooed, and feel much more self-respecting.

September 23rd. Odessa.

We four got the whole day off. It was good to be out of the crowd for a bit and the kindness of everyone, including the English colony, is indescribable. At luncheon today an old Russian lady came across the restaurant and put a great bunch of roses on our table, and a Russian officer miraculously produced some fairly recent *Graphics*. The whole town probably thinks us mad, but no matter. The papers have been heralding our arrival for some time past, and, like our own mythical Russians of 1914, the unit was seen in Odessa while it was yet tossing in the Arctic Ocean.

We ate far too much at the Petrograd Hotel, and enjoyed the opera thoroughly.

The programme of our days here is a curious one for a field hospital!

September 24th. Odessa.

Two letters after church—heavenly!

There is to be a gala performance at the opera house tonight in honour of the Grand Duchess Maria Pavlovna, an aunt of the emperor, and the mayor has invited the whole party.

Later.

We departed in trams for the opera house and found a row of beautiful boxes allotted to us. When the grand duchess arrived, they played the Russian National Anthem quite superbly. During the performance she sent a message to Dr. L, saying that she wished to inspect us, so out we had to bundle and try and look military in the foyer. When we got back the whole audience rose and stood facing our boxes while they played our National Anthem three times and cheered.

To bed about 1 completely exhausted.

September 25th. Odessa.

Dr. I. gave out at roll call that we were to leave for the Front at 6.30 this evening. It is a wonderful feeling!

The British Red Cross Unit arrives tomorrow. They are to be attached to a Serbian Division, we to another.

We got back to our old places in our old train, and the whole of the English Colony were at the station to see us off and loaded us with fruit and cigarettes.

Our destination vague.

September 26th. In the Train.

Train, and a very leisurely train. We sauntered and stopped and stopped and sauntered through Bessarabia (which is a nice name). We were let out from 4.30 to 6. A beautiful evening. The sun setting turned the dust to a flaming yellow cloud, and we found a fine church with some rather delicious singing and many paintable beggars.

It is very trying not being allowed to eat melons, I find. We aren't, because of cholera, but they are sold everywhere like potatoes, and oh! they look so good and cool, and have got lonely apricot-yellow insides.

Matron tells us we are to be in the very centre of things with Mackensen against us, and shall arrive only just in time for the push.

September 28th. In the Train.

I only know that God exists, that Love is more powerful than man, that Death can fall before us if we believe it will, that the soul of man is Power and Love. . . . I believe in God.

From *The Dark Forest.* I have been reading it all day and finished it this evening. A fine book.

September 29th. In the Train.

We arrived at Reni at 6.30 a.m., and woke to behold a pleasant stretch of river, and beyond a hazy line of hills that reminded me of Lowland Scotland. The whole morning we hung about waiting to unload, and had a very early breakfast. About 1 we took our packs down to a little passenger steamer, and about 2 began to faint with an immense internal vacuum, when we were spirited off to the Russian flagship for luncheon. We arrived to the strains of our National Anthem, thundered on a somewhat weary piano—but the sentiment's the thing! After an excellent meal, some of us were hurried off to see to the unloading of the equipment. I checked carts until 7.30 p.m. A deadly job, but the surroundings were amusing. A long quay, prisoners, Russians, Serbs, Rumanians, soldiers and sailors mounted and on foot. *Isvostchiks* (technically coachman, but used as meaning the cab of the country), country carts, Caucasians, Jews, Greeks, and Red Cross Sisters.

The Transport, with their cars, are on a barge.

Today came our first reminder of the war, the nearness of which I think we had really begun to doubt, so long has our journey been. One of the unit was hanging over the side of the boat thinking of the Danube, and the crowd, and the heat and the dust, and feeling rather weary of this disciplined globe-trotting. She was tired enough, I suppose, for things to seem a trifle purposeless—was there really going to be work to do, or were we everlastingly to chase bales and packing cases, to sightsee, to form fours and play at soldiers, in short was there really a war anywhere but on our own Western Front which was so hideously far away?

The answer came slowly, floating down the river. At first just a shapeless shadow or two which hardly attracted her attention, indeed they had almost passed before she realised that these shadows had a significance. The river was sweeping them away in a great indifference, these dead men in the blue-grey uniform of the Austrian Army.

We dined also on the flagship. Our quarters on our own boat looked altogether too grubby, so several of us slept on deck, T., B. and I in a close fat bunch for the sake of warmth. It was hard and chilly, but worth it. We left about 10.30 p.m. There is an outbreak of cholera in Galatz.

September 30th. In the Train.

We woke to sunrise, tea and biscuits, and arrived at Tchernavoda about 2, and beheld the great bridge over the Danube which carries the railway line from Constanza on to Bucharest.

We began to unload at once, and to our astonishment found an Irishman serving in the Russian Army in charge. There are two Russian infantry divisions here and one cavalry. This section of the Front is under the supreme command of a Russian General. The Russians and Serbians have borne the brunt of the fighting, and have done very well.

About 6 p.m. forty Russian soldiers turned up, and the equipment was all got off by 9. I was checking in the hold most of the time. We were bustled into a train, and left about 10, reaching Medjidia just before 11. We dozed upright in the train for the rest of the night.

CHAPTER 2

October

October 1st. Medjidia.

Woke early, and, after a scanty face and hand lick, went out for some air. Aeroplanes (our own) were circling round, the station is used as a kind of clearing hospital, and every train is either Red Cross or munitions. Otherwise a hot, dusty, uninteresting sort of place. The headquarters of the Russo-Serbian Troops. We went to breakfast at the officers' mess at 8.30. You couldn't see the food for the flies, but we were too hungry to mind. The commander-in-chief came in and made us a polite speech.

Both units are to stay here for the moment, but later Hospital B. is to move to another point 12 miles away. We are 10 miles from the firing-line, and we could hear the guns most of the morning. In the afternoon we went up to our hospital, or what is to be our hospital, and scrubbed until a party of gorgeous-looking brigands arrived who proved to be whitewashes. They have given us part of the barracks, a very good building on a hill right above the town. Next door there is a Russian Red Cross Hospital, and behind more barracks full of soldiers, dogs, puppies, pigs, cattle, and other oddments.

Went back to the train. Half the stuff is unpacked and taken up to the hospital in carts. They say there is to be heavy fighting tonight, and we are to be ready tomorrow night. We all slept in the train. I found a spare bit of floor space where anyway I could stretch. Half dead.

October 2nd. Medjidia.

Sheets of rain, and the dust is all turned to mud. And *such* mud! Off early to a breakfast of black bread and *tchi* (tea) at the Red Cross canteen, and worked at the hospital all the morning scrubbing. We are trying to fit up boilers, but so far every drop of water has to be carried from the soldiers' pump in pails. The place filthily dirty, and the sanitary (?) arrangements unspeakable.

The transport arrived tired but triumphant after an awful drive from Tchernavoda, and Mrs. M. (our cook) gave us a scrumptious tea. Worked till 8.30, and then slept chillsomely on our new camp-beds in the first-floor Ward, 75 people in one room!

Rumour says the Russians were successful in their attack last night.

October 3rd. Medjidia.

When you have time to look, or when the rain allows of your seeing anything, this place is distinctly attractive. It's fun being so high up, even though the first Bosche shell that comes this way must surely bump into the hospital. The Constanza-Tchernavoda railway runs along the valley below, and the ground sweeps up and away on the other side bare and big and brown.

The road to the Front (you wouldn't call it a road in England, but it is one really) runs past the hospital, and vanishes over the rising ground into that world of distant rumbling which is at once so suggestive and so unknown. Only some 200 yards away the old earthwork that was once Trajan's Wall lies across the *Steppe* from horizon to horizon.

We worked all day at the hospital, and by the evening the ground-floor ward for 100 patients looked really lovely. There are no beds of course, just straw mattresses laid along the floor, and empty packing cases for all furniture. But draped in a sheet even a packing case has possibilities.

By the entrance door we have rigged up a boiler and a wash-house for the lightly wounded; opposite is the secretary's room, where records of each case admitted will be kept; next door lives the disinfector, and this room is divided into two parts for the clean and dirty uniforms respectively. Then comes the ward, and on the further side the dressing-room, store-room, sterilising-room, and a wee theatre. It is the custom here to dress the wounds out of the wards as much as possible.

The Serbian general arrived late, and was amazed and enchanted. The Rumanians have fallen back, but the Russo-Serbians are moving up. We may expect men at any moment.

Sheepskins were issued to us. Just rough skins with which to line our coats. We owe this attention to the insistence of the grand duchess at Odessa.

October 4th—9th. Medjidia.

We have been working like blacks, alternately too busy and too weary to write. Men came in on Wednesday. We were at it without a break from 7.30 that morning until 1.30 on Thursday morning, then on again from 7.30 until 8.30 that night. At the end of it a mail saved our lives.

Between filth and wounds the men's condition is indescribable. They are coming back in thousands; our transport have been working absolutely heroically; and bringing the wounded in is no joke, especially at night in a strange country and over these roads.

It has been the biggest rush of wounded they have yet had. By shoving the mattresses close to each other, and putting others in every available corner, we made room for every man we could, and still the cry of the authorities was for more—more—more. In the Russian Red Cross Hospital next door two and three men were shoved on a single mattress just as they came in, the dead and the living sometimes lying side by side for hours. Even in our own wards, where British prejudice dies hard, and where every patient was in the end undressed and washed, the crawling uniforms, the dirt, the smell, the groaning men, or those still more terrible, lying in an inert silence, and last but not least the heat and the flies, made of the world a sufficiently ghastly chaos.

I don't know if the others have ever tried to imagine what coming face to face with Death would be like; I have often wondered how they took the initiation, and whether they had associated it almost inseparably, as I had, with the order and discipline of an English hospital. Something inextricably mixed up with privacy, relations, flowers, and fat black horses.

As a matter of fact, there was so much to do when the men first came in that I never gave all this a thought. One of the transport said something about a man who had died in her ambulance. I knew that several men had died on admittance, but in the wards life was the business of the moment. And then quite suddenly one of the doctors glanced over her shoulder at the man on the mattress behind her and said: "He's going, Sister." There was a quick rush and, I suppose another British prejudice, a sort of lull before they pulled the sheet over his face.

Close to me a man asked if the patient were dead. I nodded, and

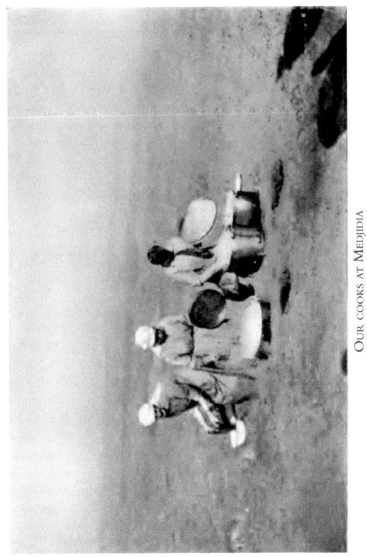

Our cooks at Medjidia

he turned and looked at the covered mattress with gentle, childlike interest. I wondered how, in this world in which he walks so familiarly, Death had still the power to make men stop and look.

Anyway, thinking was hardly possible that night, and for some time after, and by then the experience, if in no sense lighter, was at least an accepted part of the day's routine.

We have one Serbian orderly—Chris who speaks English, and "Chris, Chris, Chris! where in the world is that man? FitzRoy, go and find that man," echoes through the ward all day. And FitzRoy does go, and she finds Chris, tall and gaunt and harassed, but intensely important initiating some sufferer into the mysteries of (forgive me) a British bedpan. And from this occupation he is removed forcibly amidst piteous appeals of: "Seester, but Seester," to tell another he must lose an arm or a leg, or that a diet of black bread and sugar is not healthy if you have a bullet in your tummy, or that really the sister knows best even if she is English and mad, or that his manners are past praying for. I don't envy Chris his job, but he is very worthy. He can also walk, which is saying a lot, for our Russian orderlies can only stroll.

A shout for "Ivan "for instance, will (sometimes) produce an unclean looking individual, who beams at you down the ward with an encouraging: "*Sechas, Sestritza*" (at once, Sister), and is hurt and amazed indeed at the cries of "*Scurriscurri*" (I spell it phonetically and it means "be quick"), that pursue him day and night. They are dears, and great fun when you are *not* busy.

But in the end one does long to be able to talk oneself. All the more in a rush like this, when a dying man must be left to die for the sake of the living. What wouldn't one give to be able to help them, and to understand when they say little piteous things to one and look so sad and lonely at one's miserable: "*Ne Panemayu*" (I don't understand).

Thank Heaven we are beginning to see daylight at last; in the wards there is something approaching order, and the men who are well enough look happy and friendly.

We got a mail on the 5th. It was our last night in the top wards before we moved into tents, and was too blessed. And camp next night was wonderful. The tents are pitched on the open ground about 200 yards away from the hospital, two in each, and single ones for the officers. Below the mess tent and kitchen tent and two bath tents. The nights are chilly, but very fine and clear; you are away from the sights and sounds and smells of hospital, and there never was such a moon or such stars in all the world before. Sometimes shadowy troops singing shadowy songs move up to the Front all night; sometimes they come and camp quite close, pitching tiny canvas tents and lighting fires; always there is a flaming sunrise, and in the early morning the *steppe* looks soft and big and the town below is hidden in blue mist from the marshes.

We sound like staying here some considerable time, and they talk of getting our winter quarters ready in the barracks opposite. B. and I share a tent.

Hospital B., with a reduced staff, moves on tomorrow as a mobile field hospital. I am really glad to be in A. The others won't probably see any more of the fighting than we shall, and from the medical point of view our work will be the more interesting. Our dormitory is to be got ready for 75 new patients.

The nursing conditions are something of a revelation, but what we haven't got we invent, and what we can't invent we do without.

October 10th. Medjidia.

Hospital B. and all the transport but two moved on. There were streams of reinforcements and stuff going past us up to the Front all day, and an enemy aeroplane attacked the station. This was our first air-raid, and we were too busy even to look, though I did bolt out for a second when I was supposed to be occupying myself with something quite different. We all jumped when the first bomb went off, and then tried to look as if we hadn't! As far as we can make out we have three aeroplanes of our own here, very venerable and very slow.

There are not any trains available, so we cannot evacuate our men for a day or two. All except the desperately wounded are sent on at once when possible.

October 11th. Medjidia.

We hear there is to be a big battle in five days. Wards very hot, and the flies awful.

October 12th. Medjidia.

A very heavy day. C. came over from Hospital B. They have no work as yet.

October 13th. Medjidia.

Feeling rotten, off duty at 6. We've all had this sort of collapse, and put it down to the dust and the flies. It is impossible to keep either off the food.

October 14th. Medjidia.

I was sent to bed. A piping hot day, and we were bombarded by aeroplanes. Altogether there came twelve machines, and at times the bombardment was heavy. Two soldiers were killed in the courtyard of the hospital, but there is said to be no serious material damage. One of our own orderlies was wounded, and several civilians were brought in.

The Russians tried anti-aircraft guns, heavy guns, and machine-guns; it was all very noisy, but the aeroplanes sailed away unhurt.

October 15th. Medjidia.

Was not allowed on duty; better, but wobbly. We had one air-raid, but they lit fires all round the town so that the smoke should obscure the view.

A slack day in hospital. Our time-table:

Réveillé (a tin tray beaten by a night sister) 6.
Breakfast 7.
Roll Call and Inspection of tents 7.30
On duty 7.45
First luncheon 11.30
Second luncheon 12.30
Tea 3.15-4
Supper 8.
Off duty 3.30 to 6.30 or 12.30 to 3.30 or as much of 3 hours as possible.

The inhabitants amused themselves by burying a cholera patient in lime just below our camp this morning. Thoughtful—very!

October 16th. Medjidia.

Back on duty. The transport have brought about thirty strange tin beds from Constanza. We erected these for the worst cases, and they make a great difference—to our backs at least. They must also add to the entertainment of the "worst cases," for they have a nice little habit of collapsing at odd moments. Also they are covered with garlands of flowers and pictures of lovely ladies.

We evacuated a good number of patients, so the wards were much lighter.

October 17th. Medjidia.

Collapse of the staff. Only one sister on duty in my ward.

My birthday. We had a wonderful mail, and I received a present of chocolates when I woke up, and a further present of cigarettes and cakes was sent over from Hospital B. Mrs. M. made me a wonderful scone, and three of us picnicked happily on Trajan's Wall, watched the aeroplanes, and tried to ignore the unavoidable proximity of a decomposing horse. It was a very nice birthday indeed.

October 18th. Medjidia.

We had an awful night, as the wind arose, and twice B. and I had to sally forth in our pyjamas to hammer in tent pegs and rescue the kitchen stove. The three bath tents were blown flat, and most of the mess and kitchen tents blown away.

October 19th. Medjidia.

A bad aeroplane raid at Hospital B., and they were bringing in wounded civilians to us all day. Ghastly. The flash of the guns at night is very clear now, and the sound continuous. Our 1st Serbian division has done splendidly, but has been so cut up it has been withdrawn, and for the winter we shall be nursing Russians. Some of the Cossacks of the Imperial Guard camped here for the day, and troops streamed up to the line without a pause.

We have erected a "Sick" tent for the staff. Hospital B. and the transport sent over their invalids.

October 20th. Medjidia.

An aeroplane bombarded us in the morning, and the guns are very clear.

As I went on duty after tea there came a message from the Serbian Headquarters ordering us to evacuate all our men at once and to follow ourselves in twenty-four hours. The news came as rather a shock, and we got the men off sadly enough. Later we were visited by the Russian commander-in-chief, who told us it was true the army had fallen back, but that we and the Russian Red Cross Hospital were all he had to depend on and the wounded pouring in. So of course Dr. I. said we'd stay only too thankfully. Our superfluous equipment is to be sent to Constanza by train, and we are to work as a field dressing station and evacuate (if it becomes necessary) with the army. There is a rumour that the line to Tchernavoda is cut. The bridge has been hit by a bomb, but not irreparably damaged.

A tiny mail wandered in in the evening.

October 21st. Medjidia.

The Russian Hospital left. We spent a long day packing and getting the stores off. They are to go to Galatz, as Constanza is not now considered sufficiently safe. We struck camp, and all the men were evacuated, though a good many new cases passed through to be dressed on their way back from the Front. These were mostly walking cases, as the more serious are now sent farther back. But it was interesting work dressing these weary men who had toiled in on their own for the most part.

I went twice down to the station with the baggage in the evening, a perilous journey in rickety carts, through pitch darkness over roads (?), crammed with troops and refugees, which were lit up periodically by the most amazing green lightning I have ever seen, and the roar and flash of the guns was incessant. At the station no lights were allowed because of enemy aircraft, but the place was illuminated here and there by the camp fires of a new Siberian Division which had just arrived. Picked troops these and magnificent men.

We wrestled with the baggage until 2 a.m., and went back to the hospital in one of our own cars. One orderly came in almost in tears. Her cart had twice turned over completely on its way to the station, so on arrival she had hastened to Dr. I. a tale of woe and a scratched face.

Dr. I. said: "That's right, dear child, that's right, *stick* to the equipment." Which may very well be described as the motto of the unit these days!

I dropped on to a mattress in the ward just as I was, as we may have to leave ourselves at 5. Six of the unit are to accompany the equipment to Galatz, but mercifully I am not one of them.

October 22nd. Medjidia—Saragea.

We were woken at 4.30, and breakfasted on a small bit of bread and butter and *tchi*. There were no orders from headquarters and the guns were incessant and sounded nearer. We spent a lazy morning, and about luncheon time got orders to evacuate at once. The majority are to go to Galatz by train with Dr. C., the rest (self included) are to go by road with Dr. I. and work with the army as a clearing station.

The train party got off as quick as possible, and about 4 a big lorry came for our equipment. We loaded it, seven of us mounted on the top, and the rest went in two of our own cars. The scene was really intensely comic. Seven Scottish Women balanced precariously on the pile of luggage, a Serbian Doctor, with whom Dr. I. is to travel, standing alongside in an hysterical condition, imploring us to hurry, telling

38

us the Bulgarians were as good as in the town already, Dr. I. quite un-moved demanding the whereabouts of the Ludgate Boiler, somebody arriving at the last minute with a huge open barrel of treacle, which, of course, could not possibly be left to a German—oh dear, how we laughed!

At last we started with orders to make for Carlo Murat. In the town our driver took us out of our way to pick up an officer, and in so do-ing we missed the others, who thought we were on ahead. The road to Carlo Murat proved to be only mud and quite impossible for a heavy lorry after the rain, so we had to give up the idea of getting there and decided to push on to the Military Headquarters at Saragea.

We heard later that Medjidia fell the afternoon after we left.

The whole country is in retreat, and we had an extraordinarily interesting drive. Behind we could see the shells exploding, and the sky was alight with the glow of burning villages. On our right a big-ger glow showed the fate of Constanza, which fell today. The road was indescribably dilapidated, and crammed with refugees, troops, and transport. The retreating troops seem mostly Rumanian; I gather the Russians are protecting our rear.

The peasants are a picturesque lot, not of course purely Rumanian, as the Dobrudja was so lately a Turkish province. Ponies and oxen are harnessed into their little springless carts, all their household goods are packed inside, and they are followed by terrified flocks of sheep, pigs, and cattle. The peasants trudge along, going—one wonders where?

It was showery at first, but turned to a beautiful night though very dark. Our progress was slow, as the lamp refused to burn, but we cheered the way with frugal rations of biscuits, jam, and cheese. Though lost we have at least had the intelligence to get lost with the food!

We reached Saragea about 10.30, almost too tired to speak, our lorry deposited us in the mud by the roadside, bade us a tender fare-well—and left. But the general of division was very kind, invited us into headquarters and refreshed us with black bread and *tchi*. We ate amidst a chaos of maps, generals, messengers, and field telephones. The men looked anxious to breaking-point, but their kindness to seven lone females is unforgettable. Our kit they stuck under a form of shelter in charge of a sentry, and we groped our way through deep, deep mud to a house where we were given two rooms. Mud floors, hard but clean.

October 23rd. Hirsovar.

We scraped the surface dirt off our hands in filthy water, and then set out in search of news and breakfast. The endless procession of troops and refugees never ceased to tramp past all night, and there was no news of the unit. Meanwhile the general had sent to Hirsovar, on the Danube (I think a distance of about 60 kilometres), for two lorries to fetch us and our stuff. A very nice Russian boy gave us boiling water and half a loaf in exchange for treacle and cigarettes; P., I rather fear, looted four eggs, which we hard boiled, and so breakfasted handsomely. The rest of the morning we spent dealing out treacle. The soldiers very soon discovered it, and fell out as they marched past, bringing everything, down to their water-bottles, in which to carry it away. About 11 Dr. I. and three of our transport cars drove up. Having invented every awful fate for us, her relief was immense when she found us sitting by the roadside drinking Bovril. Orders to evacuate at once came to the village, and the staff moved off.

It was a pretty heart-breaking sight to watch the people stripping their little houses and packing what they could into some tiny cart. The women sobbing, and the men dogged and inert. Here and there on the road, of course, there were moments of panic in which they lost all self-control. Men, at the cry that the Bulgars were coming, dragged women and children out of carts so as to make good their own escape, and would even in their terror fling their own babies down on the roadside when these hampered them. I wish that certain people living securely in a certain island could see a country in retreat—not an army only, but a whole country, women and children and beasts—it's not a pretty sight, but it's a very fine lesson.

The transport were sent off at once, but Dr. I. insisted on staying with us until the arrival of the lorries. Our orders are to reach Galatz *via* Hirsovar and the Danube, and there report to the consul. Dr. I. proceeds with the Serbian Hospital. We waited several hours until the stream of troops had got considerably thinner, and only isolated soldiers straggled by with varying reports as to the nearness of the enemy. One rumour said their cavalry was only three miles away—and this to my mind is quite sufficiently near. The 8th Army has arrived to strengthen our left flank, our right at Tchernavoda is safe for the present.

At last Captain B. passed by in a car, and got out to speak to us. He managed to commandeer a passing lorry, and by 4 o'clock we had packed in ourselves and the equipment, and bidden farewell to Dr.

I., who was proceeding in one of our own cars by a rather different route.

We found ourselves at the mercy of an insane driver, who dashed along regardless of anybody, wrecked one refugees' cart, terrified the horses all along the road, and stopped for nothing and nobody. As Captain B. had had to knock him down twice before the poor little man would consent to take us at all he no doubt thought here was a great chance of getting his own back. At last at dusk he charged a cart, made a belated attempt to avoid it, and drove clean over the edge of the road. Luckily for us the embankment happened to be low at that point. We climbed down and after much heaving and struggling some soldiers got the car on the road again.

A little later we came to the edge of the high ground and in the distance far below us saw the river glistening. It was pitch dark, and our only lamp refused to work, though this in no wise affected our headlong career. The next thing we nearly slaughtered was a Rumanian officer in an Isvostchik. After that in the interest of the public safety I sat aloft with my electric torch, and we hurtled on by its none too brilliant light. Our driver tipped us off the road once more, but finally landed us at headquarters at Hirsovar, shattered but alive. Here again the Russians were very kind. First they took us to supper at a Red Cross canteen, and then two officers turned out of their rooms in our favour. We got hold of a puddle of hot water, and fell to the floor in contented heaps.

October 24th. Hirsovar—Galatz.

The general called us at 4.30 a.m. in person, to enable us to catch a boat for Galatz. In the end we had a long wait, and the opportunity of watching a delicious sunrise over the Danube. A party of Rumanian officers, still very ' well dressed,' refreshed us with *tchi*.

As we sat at our little iron tables outside the restaurant, with our lovely glasses of deep amber *tchi*, and heaps and heaps of sugar, down the road came the weary, muddy figure of a soldier. With a cry of "David," we all simultaneously leapt to our feet. It was our laundry orderly from Medjidia. The poor old fellow had lost the others, had walked all the way, and had quite, quite given up hope of ever seeing us again. He was too touchingly happy for words at finding us.

After considerable difficulty we all got put on a barge with our equipment in immediate succession to a regiment of cavalry. The condition of the deck was awful. They crowded on a whole army of wounded, Rumanian and Serb, the worst cases on wooden shelves below deck with not a soul to look after them, and the rest strewn about on the filthy upper deck with soaking bandages and not even a bench to sit on. We did what we could, but it was not much, and found a fairly clean spot where we camped, and where S. improvised the most wonderful meals. Mercifully it did not rain, and the afternoon was clear and beautiful. We left about 10 a.m. and they landed us on a Russian Hospital Ship at Galatz about 9 this evening.

The little sisters looked far too beautiful to be really hard worked, but for the moment to look beautiful seemed the more essential, and the officers who all spoke French were charming. While the sailors landed that something equipment they took us in, gave us water to wash in and a delicious meal. They were optimistic as to eventual success, but spoke very bitterly of the slaughter and suffering the retreat had entailed. But, of course, one must not forget that the Rumanians had a very stiff time of it for any army, let alone an untried one, and no artillery to speak of.

Ambulances from the British Red Cross Hospital here were sent to fetch us, and we went off to the hospital, where we found Dr. C. and all the train party, including B., who had saved the equipment and generally covered herself with glory. We spent the night all together in a tent on the hard, damp ground—a most bitter disappointment!

October 25th. Galatz.

Galatz is big and middling dull—but boasts a very fine cake shop, where we lived most of the day—when we weren't washing—enjoying a very unwarlike diet. Four of us got leave to sleep out, and took rooms in an hotel. We had one heavenly night of sheets, with coffee and rolls for *déjeuner* in the morning.

A rumour is abroad to the effect that Tchernavoda has fallen, but that the bridge has been destroyed.

October 26th. Galatz.

J. and I went up to the British Red Cross Hospital to see if we could do anything to help, and were repulsed, along with all the sisters! Mrs. H. arrived. The transport, except for the five reported to be with Dr. I., are all safe at Braila, and Miss H. with three others turned up here later. Rumour says that Hospital B. is safe with the Serbian Hospital, and that Dr. I. is still at Hirsovar, working at a dressing station at the request of the Rumanians. The town has been evacuated.

I went into the wards after tea—work very heavy.

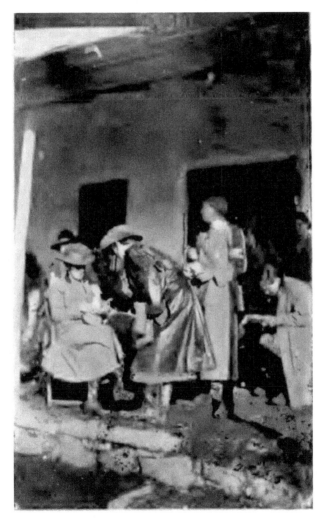

Dr. Inglis at Saragea

A charming black terrier, with a white shirt front, has adopted us.

October 27th. Galatz.

Worked in the wards most of the day—heaps to do and rather terrible. The patients are all Rumanian.

There is great talk of a general evacuation from here.

October 28th. Braila.

Dr. I. turned up directly after breakfast. She is safely at Braila with the rest, and reports Hospital B. to be at Reni. I was in the wards at 8.30, and about 10.30 J. came to fetch me, and we went down to the quay to rescue some stores the British Red Cross are lending us. The greater part of their equipment is being sent back to Odessa.

Nearly all our nursing staff are to go forward to Braila. I hurled a few things into a rug, and just caught the boat. Braila is about an hour's journey up the river, and Dr. C. is in charge, as Dr. I. has gone to Reni for a day or two to see Hospital B. I had tea, and saw C., who is working hard in a Rumanian Hospital, as is every member of the transport who has had any nursing experience. Six of us went off after supper and worked until 2 a.m. at a dressing-station. Some lovely ladies were hovering around when we arrived. I'm afraid we turned them out.

It was good for the work, even if it was bad for the entente! Wounded were lying about on the floors of five or six rooms in their uniforms without so much as a mattress. They could mostly move a little by themselves, and everyone to whom it was possible proceeded to crawl, hop, or wriggle into the dressing-room. We carried in one or two who were helpless, but only the cases that really needed attention. The rest just slept, and slept, and slept, as if they could never be deep enough asleep.

We are told they have 11,000 wounded here, and only 7 doctors.

Got back to the consulate about done. We had no baggage, so we lay down on the floor as we were. Very good news from Verdun.

October 29th. Braila.

Most of the transport went off early to Galatz. C. remains to drive Dr. I. I went to the Rumanian Hospital with her, but found a lull in the rush, so went back to the consulate and got a sleep in someone else's bed. After supper, J. and I went to a Rumanian Hospital on our own, and put in some work under a very nice Rumanian doctor. Dr. I. returned, and we moved into our new quarters. We have been given quite an attractive little house by the authorities, though it possesses

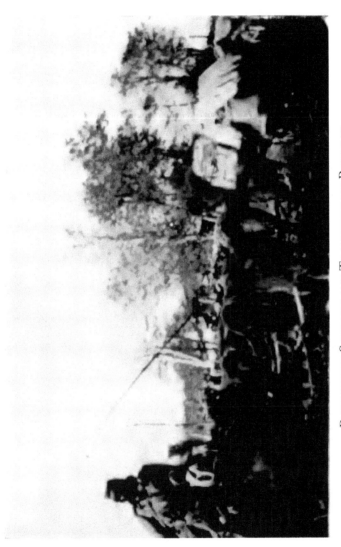

ROUMANIAN SOLDIERS AND TRANSPORT ON RETREAT

real drains, which is a trifle bewildering! All the rooms open on to a passage, which in its turn gives on to a courtyard, round two sides of which the house is built. Lovely beds, and for the first time for weeks we slept like tops.

October 30th. Braila.

M., J., and I went back to the hospital, where we find our talents are highly appreciated! It is really nothing but a huge dressing-station, and some of the male students that work there are devils and torture the men quite unnecessarily. After supper we had our second cholera inoculation. I spent a horrid nightmary night. Crowds and crowds of wounded were pouring in, and I could neither move nor help. That particular dream is becoming a habit, and I don't like it.

October 31st. Braila.

Felt extremely ill all day! Our hospital opened; it includes one floor in a Rumanian Hospital, with dressing-room and theatre, besides another big dressing-station a little way off.

The Rumanian Army is said to have been sent to the Carpathians, but of this there is no official confirmation.

I haven't changed my clothes since we fled—disgusting!

CHAPTER 3

November

November 1st. Braila.

In the wards and lots doing. In mine there are over 60 patients (Rumanians), and all the windows are tight shut! They are unattractive, complaining creatures, with very little self-control, but one is profoundly sorry for them. A few have fine physique, of a Latin type, but I am told and can well believe that phthisis is a terrible scourge in the country. In peace time they live amongst miserable surroundings, and are ground down by the Jews.

The town is quite amusing, and there is a perfectly excellent *café*—the Français—run by an old Italian, who used to be at a big hotel in Paris, and apparently a close friend of King Edward. He loves C. quite devotedly; we go there together, and he cooks us a wonderful little supper all to ourselves. There is also a picture palace, to which I have not yet been, an amusing peasants' market, and a Persian shop with beautiful rugs and carpets. I have already begun to desire riches once more!

November 2nd. Braila.

Colder, and a rumour that our kit bags will arrive tomorrow.

November 3rd. Braila.

A small mail. Work is getting slack, and the atmosphere in the Wards is something excruciating. We carry on an open-air campaign under hideous difficulties.

Today six of us moved down to the consulate to relieve the crowd at the cottage. C. and I share a bed, and are very happy. The consul has fallen ill elsewhere, so the other four are luxuriously spread over the drawing-room.

Our kit bags arrived—oh, such good, clean, clean clothes.

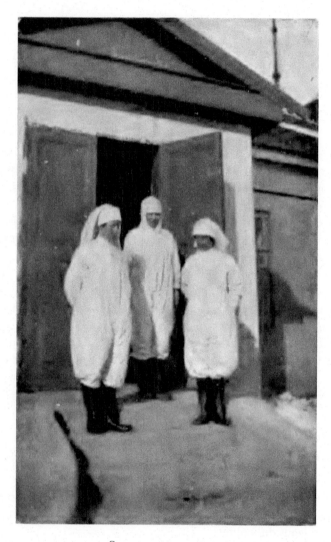

Sisters in typhus kit

November 8th. Braila.

Work as usual and quite busy. I begin to like my patients a little better! Went to the theatre in the evening to help with a perfectly filthy leg amputation.

November 9th. Braila.

I dined with C. at the Français tonight, and after dinner we slipped down to the river in the car. Such a heavenly night, and it all looked so kind and peaceful.

November 10th. Braila.

A busy day *in* the ward and two men died. Various Russians from General Headquarters came to tea. Apparently the Rumanians failed to blow up the bridge at Tchernavoda, but they hope to hold the enemy on the Constanza-Tchernavoda line until some heavy artillery from England gets out. Should Kola be kept open they may continue to advance this winter, but if the port is frozen and unavailable they will have to wait until May. Meanwhile it is said that the Serb Division will re-form somewhere near Reni.

November 12th. Braila.

A *huge* mail! Too thrilled and delighted for words, and it is all good news. I am even now sitting up in bed, clad in all the splendour of a new jersey sent by Mother, and which distracts my attention quite dreadfully, just because it is so nice to be wearing something really attractive—and so comfortable.

November 13th. Braila.

Work as usual. Our names have all been taken by the Russian commander-in-chief for decoration for the Medjidia affair. What fun!

November 14th. Braila.

After supper I went down to the Monopol to have coffee with X., and found her surrounded by a strange crowd of Russian and Greek civilians. They were most polite. The Greek next to me was a Turkish subject, but had left Constantinople at the outbreak of war so as to avoid serving in their army. A party of Russian officers dining at a table near by insisted on our joining them while they drank a health to England. They were charming. A glass to every toast is the rule here—so I left early!

November 18th. Braila.

Usual day and very cold. We have orders to give up the fresh-air campaign, as we were almost imperilling international relations thereby, so the wards are something indescribable.

I am told that the great provision difficulty is partly due to the cholera, as the country people are afraid to bring their stuff into the town.

November 20th. Braila.

An air-raid, the first since we left Medjidia. It was a gorgeous day, and I went for a long walk.

November 21st. Braila.

The war news from the Transylvanian Front is not good. Commander Locker-Lampson and his armoured cars are said to be in or near Braila. They had to leave the Caucasus, as the roads were impossible.

(*Extract from a letter.*)

Nothing can beat the tales about us in Odessa. I enclose one cutting—but the best story tells of how the Scottish Women leapt into the sea at Constanza so as to escape the pursuing Bulgar!

We are very busy again in hospital now, and no sign of moving. You will hardly believe it credible, but I am the one who rises first at the consulate and calls the rest! C. has gone back to the Transport Headquarters, a two days' journey, where they are kicking their heels with fury, and have nothing to do. The other hospital, too, is slack, so we give ourselves horrid airs.

(*Extract from an Odessa paper referred to above.*)

Rumanian refugees arriving from Medjidia tell about the work of the British Women's Hospital. Immediately upon their arrival they arranged an exemplary hospital for 200 beds. The unit divided, and a part of the nurses went to the nearest firing-line; the Rumanians call the work of the British women ideal, and in fact the fearlessness and energy of the British women is beyond praise. Four British nurses of the transport stayed in Medjidia till the last moment, picking up the wounded soldiers, and taking them back.

When the foe got hold of Medjidia, the British women had scarcely time to jump into their motors and go out of the town. The Rumanian Army and convoy were already out of sight and the British women had to stray in the mountains in abandoned places without knowledge of country or food three days. Nevertheless, they forced their way on to the good roads, and in three days came to Reni. The first thing they asked of Admiral Vosselkin, who heartily met them there, was to give them a bath, and only after a good wash in the Russian baths they asked for food. They were given a good meal, and taken to Galatz.

November 23rd. Braila.

The wounded are pouring in, but are mostly moderate cases from the Transylvania Front.

Our newest rumour: We are all to be shipped to Salonica *via* Kola. God forbid!

November 24th. Braila.

Meat rations failed. A busy day. Francis Joseph is dead.

November 25th. Braila.

We had tea at a neighbouring hospital this evening. Most of the Rumanian girls in these hospitals seem very young, but are amazingly self-confident for their years. And for all their emotionalism the real horror of it seems to miss them entirely. They like physical horrors in a sense, for the sake of the sensation, or so it would seem. Of course this particular town is far from being representative, and has a large preponderance of elements, Greek and Jewish.

We have very bad news from both Fronts, and Bucharest is being evacuated. The Rumanians can only put 1,000,000 men all told into the field, and they are mostly peasants taken away from the vital work on the land. For the last two years the army has been concentrated at intervals, first at one point then at another, with the result that stores of grain have been left unsown for want of labour, and these stores will make rich booty for the Germans if they fall into their hands.

We are very busy, 7,000 wounded in the town.

Still no rations.

November 26th. Braila.

Everyone hideously depressed, and the government has moved to Jassi.

One feels desperately sorry for these people, with the lesson of Serbia and Belgium before them. Since the junction at Ploesti fell they seem to have lost heart with a rush. The country, with all its enormous stores of oil and grain, is just being abandoned to the enemy. The line to be held is roughly drawn from the southwest boundary of Moldavia through the north of the Dobrudja. The latter Front has been handed over entirely to the Russians.

Our plans are more settled. Hospital B. is to remain with the Serbs at Ismail, and we are to take over a Russian Hospital at Issacea in the Dobrudja. The transport are to work farther south between us and Babadagh.

Here an endless flow of wounded. We put some of the beds together, and the men three in two beds, but even then had not enough room. It is the same everywhere. You see groups of hungry, weary men crowding the pavement before every hospital.

I was told of a Rumanian artist today who lives in Bucharest and does strange subconscious drawings—rather in the manner of Planchette—a power he has possessed for six years. After the war he intends coming to London.

November 27th. Braila.

Two Russian sisters have been attached to the unit, one to Hospital A., one to the Transport Section, to act as interpreters and to keep the Russian accounts. They are at least very decorative members of the community.

November 28th. Braila.

No news. Rumour in this land of rumour says that letters will soon be difficult either to send or to receive.

CHAPTER 4

December

December 1st. Braila.

Work as usual; colder.

News from Bucharest says that the enemy have been pushed back 20 miles, and there are excellent, though vague, accounts of good work in the Dobrudja. Still no mail.

December 3rd. Braila.

A small mail, but it was absolutely thrilling.

December 4th. Braila.

(Extract from a letter.)

Our plans are once more changed. The transport have gone to Babadagh as before arranged, Hospital B. goes back with the Serbs to some place near Odessa, and we are being sent forward to Ciulnitza on the main line between Tchernavoda and Bucharest. We move the day after tomorrow, and are frightfully pleased. The news is better, and rumour has it that the oilfields have been destroyed, which I hope is true.

There has been lots of work here, but the people are rather odious. They say our hospital is run entirely by German Jews, so perhaps it is not surprising that we do not hit it off completely. The real Rumanians have been charming to us; the women are very good-looking.

J. and I gave such a successful tea-party the other day in honour of the birthdays of our respective sisters. We pinched some wood from the house, lit a fire at the consulate, and entertained a party of seven to tea and supper. The guests came at 4.30 and stayed until 10, and we all agreed we had enjoyed nothing so much for three months. Of course we sat in the firelight, and told ghost stories. The consul's two little Rumanian maids rose to the occasion, and when we got back from the Wards we found a beautiful English table spread with the consul's best china and silver and nothing forgotten, not even ash-trays and a cigarette-box. It only wanted a mail to make things perfect.

December 5th. Braila.

We nearly had a real pogrom in the wards this evening. Earlier in the day the Jew secretary had told one of the patients that this war would wipe all the nations off the face of Europe, and leave the Jews the masters of the world. This evening he came upstairs on business, and the moment he appeared the patient leapt out of bed, beat upon his plate with a spoon, and delivered an impassioned address. The Jew was very nearly torn to pieces on the spot, and I found my sympathies were at the time distinctly Christian!

We took a fond farewell of the men whom we really do like more than we thought possible at first. J. goes back to Hospital B. tomorrow, so we went and had a farewell *café* at the Français. There we found some English flying men. They had flown from Imbros to Bucharest, and had been ordered away from Ciulnitza only this morning!

December 6th. In the Train.

Packed. We are only to take bed-bundles with us, which is rather a relief, as I gather we are bound to retreat before very long. We got into our train about 7 p.m. It consists of one coach and one truck for the equipment, so five of us arranged to sleep with and on the latter. It was a quaint scene when we had all settled down, but we made ourselves quite comfortable on the bales and we wrapped everything we possessed round and round us.

We are reunited to our old Medjidia orderlies, and have twenty-five of them with us at the moment. .

(*Extract from a letter.*)

By now we orderlies are wily folk. We know how travelling in "furrin" parts affects the unit, and decided that being on our own would compensate amply for being cold. So five of us volunteered to share the truck, and it was once a German truck, with the equipment. I was in one attic, that is on our topmost layer of bales under the roof, our secretary reposed on the next ledge just below me, M. our anaesthetist was flung recklessly across space in the laundry trough, and the two others lay in state on camp beds on our limited floor space. There were no windows, so for the sake of light the door had to be open by day and it froze hard just after we started. Wednesday night we slept in the train. It was somewhat disturbed and chilly, and we did not leave

OUR SANITARS

Braila until 8 on Thursday morning.

About 10 we made ourselves an excellent breakfast of *tchi*, bread, sardines, and chocolate. The weather was very cold, and we kept going most of the time across a desolate flat landscape. All day we improvised excellent meals (a distracting amount of chocolate was produced), and we danced breakdowns at intervals to keep warm. Reached Ciulnitza about 5. It is nothing but a large station full of wandering rumours to the effect that Bucharest has fallen, and that our being allowed to stay is uncertain.

Dr. I. had us all out to sleep in a sort of waiting room place. In the middle of the night I had reason to suspect, and by morning had acquired proof that I had merely slipped into a bed (bedclothes and all), that had but lately been vacated by a Russian soldier. So had B. However, the consequences might have been worse and it was quite the funniest night I have ever spent. Half the soldiers in the place had apparently been accustomed to live there, and so would burst in at odd moments to fetch their belongings. B. was next the door, and it was her business to prevent them—if she could—so, whenever I opened an eye, there she was capering about the room in her pyjamas, pursuing some bewildered foreigner, and shouting: "*Idé—idé* (Go, go)—oh, you fool, why don't you go, *Idé, idé*," while the unit howled with mirth and Dr. I. vainly tried to .assert a sense of outraged propriety.

December 8th. In the Train.

Breakfasted at 8, after which Dr. I. went off to search for the authorities. We walked up to the aerodrome, and found five small French machines and three big English just arrived. They all had orders to evacuate at once. Bucharest has fallen, all communications are therefore cut, and the army is falling back and will take up this position tomorrow.

Back to the station for luncheon. Food is running very low. Dr. I. announced that our orders were to leave. What wounded they are able to move are being taken farther back.

The Russian Red Cross people at Braila can have known very little of the situation up here. We are to go back to Ciura. So we packed ourselves once more into our truck, and watched the aeroplanes depart. They looped the loop over our train, and waved farewell. We had orders not to leave our carriages, and news came through that everyone was to be out of the place before 5, as the station would then be destroyed. So we spent the afternoon watching train after train, each with its crowd of refugees and soldiers, creep away. At 5 to 5 it was almost dark, we were still lying in the station, and eight trucks of explosives had just been hooked on.

A young and quite presentable Rumanian officer had been helping us to open our methylated barrel for cooking purposes, when huge flames were seen leaping up alongside our engine. He dashed forward to see what was happening, and instantly the place became a seething mass of jumping, screaming humanity. The officer came running back, shouting to us to shut the truck doors. We hauled him in, and slid the door to. It must have been touch and go to take our train with its load of "*obus*" within a few inches of what proved to be a blazing oil-tank. As soon as our carriage was past, we got the door open again. The horizon was in a blaze, oil-tanks, granaries, straw-stacks, everything burnable was set light to. It was very terrible and very beautiful. Peasants, men, women, and children were running alongside the train in a panic, trying to clamber into the already overcrowded trucks, others had given up the struggle, and collapsed by the side of the line, or had settled down into that familiar dogged tramp with the blazing sky behind them.

The officer came as far as Slovosia with us. By rights, it is an hour's journey, but we took three. Our guest was really interesting and quite tolerant and intelligent. The great hope of the Rumanian Army was, he said, General Avarescu, who gave up the command in the Dobrudja before the fall of Constanza, in order to take the supreme command in the Carpathians.

We gave our guest supper. Soup, bread and cheese, bread and sugar, bread and sardines, chocolate and cigarettes, the last of our private supplies, but all, we felt, in a good cause.

December 9th. In the Train.

I slept very well, and M. got up and gave us all breakfast at 10. We waited most of the morning for the train to go on, and by 3.30 were approaching Tanderei (the junction where the line to Braila branches off from the main line to Tchernavoda), and feeling very bored and cold when I saw an aeroplane planing down towards us. She was hovering quite low, and apparently just over our engine, when we heard a loud explosion, and realised she must be German. The whole place became alive with soldiers. The enemy followed up with a smart machine-gun fire; the French officer, who was travelling with Dr. L, leapt out of his carriage, shouting: "*Tirez, tirez, donc!*" and two more loud explosions followed. We made one dash for the bales to try and find bandages and dressings, the Russian Army remembered their rifles, and the aeroplane was driven off. In the station we found that the material damage was small, and the casualties only one horse killed and two men wounded. The aeroplane returned, and dropped two more bombs, but was driven off easily.

Our engine-driver felt so shattered that he actually hastened our departure, and we went much comforted by a drink of hot soup provided by some Russian sisters.

We did not reach Ciura until 10.30 p.m. and then only to discover it had been evacuated at midday, and that we were to go on and try our luck at Faurei.

December 10th. In the Train.

Woke up after rather a miserable night, as my packing cases had got disorganised. The world very cold and rather hungry. At some wayside station Dr. I. found a goose, a duck, a hen, and half a pig. Our Russki's cooked them for us, the pork not half bad, and we got a liberal supply of bread and sugar. Last night's storm of wind and rain has abated, but it froze hard, and this morning the world was a big waste adorned by icicles. The water is pea-green, and has to be boiled for ten minutes, but the Russian Red Cross people again came to the rescue with soup. We move infinitesimal distances at long intervals, and are told we are just about to get into the congestion! Saw a long column of artillery retreating across the plain. All tucked up by 8 p.m.

December 11th. In the Train.

A very cold night, but the truck woke in excellent spirits, and we had good *tchi* for breakfast. After that we got into the saltmarsh district, and could get nothing but salt water, which was misery. Reached Faurei soon after 1, and found nothing there but mud, trains, and orders to go on to Braila. All the trucks from the north come in covered in snow.

Arrived late at Braila.

December 12th. Braila.

We woke in a siding to brilliant sunshine. B. and I went up to the town early. The water supply is off, so there are no baths to be had—rather a blow, as I have not moved out of my clothes from my fur coat downwards for five days.

At the Russian Headquarters Dr. I. was told that we should probably proceed to Traian, some 25 kilometres in the direction of Faurei, there to work as a dressing-station.

B. and I met Colonel Griffiths, the Head of the British Oil Destroying Mission, and he lent us his room at the Français for the afternoon. It was rather fun, as the officers of his staff were running in and out all the time, and were very interesting. It seems that everything now depends upon holding the railway junction at Buzei, east of Ploesti, where the lines from Braila and Moldavia meet. The Germans are making a big offensive movement there, and it is just a chance whether or no the Russians will arrive in time to hold it. The loss of the line will probably mean the evacuation of Braila and Galatz.

Many tons of grain have fallen to the Germans, but, thanks to the British Mission, no oil.

At tea we heard that owing to the serious news from the Front our departure was to be delayed, and meanwhile the Russian authorities had provided us with two empty rooms in which to sleep. They are in a house perched on the cliff above the Danube, with a heavenly view. We got out camp beds and bundles, and passed a decidedly chilly night.

I heard a most pathetic description today of the funeral of the Queen of Rumania's little son in the Royal Chapel at Bucharest. And a curious thing happened just before the child died. He nearly always spoke English, but, at the end, after having been unconscious for a considerable time, he suddenly said in Rumanian: "It is finished." He was only three.

December 13th. Braila.

Grey and wet. The streets inches deep in liquid mud. After tea Dr. I. announced that the Buzei line was not to be held, and in consequence we are to start work at Galatz and leave tomorrow. Glad at least to have something settled.

I got some hot water out of the other inhabitants of our villa, and we went to bed very clean and happy.

December 14th. Braila.

Heard definitely after tea that the congestion on the line was too great to allow of our going today, then hardly had we got back to the house and erected the beds than an order came that we were to go at once. Packed in a fearful hurry, and went down to the station. There we sat in a waiting-room full of officers from 5 p.m. to 5 a.m. Quite the most appalling night I have ever spent. At last the train turned up from the port, and I tumbled into the truck.

December 15th. In the Train.

We woke soon after 9 to find ourselves just outside Braila, and spent the whole day in the train crawling along at intervals. At about 7.30 p.m. we arrived at Barbosi, and the commandant of the station gave us an excellent meal of potatoes cooked in oil. A Rumanian officer, on his way to the Front with stores, contributed some tinned meat. He and a friend paid their respects to Dr. I., and then visited us in the truck and stayed until 11. They made lovely Turkish coffee, and told us the story of their lives, which was—dramatic! We all parted sworn friends.

December 16th. Galatz.

Reached Galatz about 5 a.m., 15 miles in 36 hours! A tiny mail awaited us, but it was good to get. Spent the rest of the day getting clean. I am billeted in a dear little house with five of the others. Sambo, our terrier, is here. He was with the Transport for a time, then returned to Galatz with a Hospital B. Orderly. He is the most perfect gentleman I have ever met.

December 17th. Galatz.

Roll call at 9 a.m. It is said that we are to start a hospital here 2 miles outside the forts, but no definite arrangement has yet been come to. Matron goes to Odessa by boat to-night with the greater part of the equipment. B. and I went down to help and worked on the quay until 9.30. Beautiful night. An endless stream of guns and ammunition going up to the forts from the quay and the news from the Front very bad.

December 18th. Galatz.

Today I have never stopped walking for a moment. The Russians are evacuating all their own hospitals, and we have got to go too. The enemy are already this side of Faurei, and are threatening Braila. I spent the afternoon and evening getting stores. Where, when, and how we go is uncertain. We could hear the guns today, and the station was a seething mass of refugees all fighting to get on the platform— everything guarded by sentries.

December 19th. Galatz.

Did stores from 8.30 a.m. until 6 p.m. Hospital B. is to evacuate to Odessa tonight with the British Red Cross Unit. We are to stay here. The Russians say they will not take the responsibility of getting us away, but nevertheless would like us to stay. Am glad.

December 20th. Galatz.

A Russian success is reported between Faurei and Braila, and four guns taken. This evening huge guns passed us on their way up from the quay to the town defences, some parts drawn by teams of not less than twelve oxen.

December 21st. Galatz.

Our hostess's son told us that Mr. Asquith has resigned, and that Lloyd George has formed a ministry. Most exciting, and we are longing for the English papers. The news from the Front continues to be good.

Patriotism must be a difficult problem out here. Our hosts are of Greek birth, but were for many years Turkish subjects, with interests in both Constantinople and Asia Minor. For a considerable time now they have lived at Galatz. This son has a Greek passport, and of his three brothers one is interned as a Turkish subject, another is in Bucharest with a Spanish passport, where the third was killed the other day in an air-raid. Of the two sons-in-law one is a Turkish subject exiled at Salonica; the other, also a Turkish subject, fought for the Russians through the siege of Port Arthur, and is now interned at Constantinople as a Russian Officer.

They are very frightened, poor people. We were sitting in our little room today and writing letters when *Madame* entered, her face all white and flabby, and said solemnly: "*Boom—boom.*" At first we thought it was a joke, but, no, it wasn't; it was an air-raid! But the old lady must find considerable consolation for these and other fortunes of war in the vast sums she is making out of the Scottish Women for our billets!

The house is wee, and there are two beds between five of us. So two have migrated to sofas next door. B. and I spent one woeful night together, and I've now retired to a mattress on the floor and am very comfortable. But what we really enjoy are our suppers. The Russians give us an allowance of 2 *lei* (2 *frs.*) per head per day, so instead of being economical at some restaurant, we pool our allowances, and have wonderful and exclusive feasts here. And the market is most attractive, and far bigger than the one at Braila.

December 22nd. Galatz.

I went for a long walk with B., and we found a large and beautiful lake north of the town. It was delicious, all blue and sparkly, with little boats dipping about in it.

There is a rumour that Tultcha has fallen, but it is, I believe, untrue. On the contrary, so says our host: "*Les Russes ont détruit les Bulgares et les ont jetés dans un lac!*"

December 23rd. Galatz.

A telegram came from Iliatchenko, the chief of the Russian Red Cross, ordering the British Red Cross Unit to move at once. They leave tonight, and the greater part of our equipment, including our kit-bags, is to go with them to Odessa.

We visited our new hospital. It is in a dark and dismal slum between the port and the station. We slithered through much mud and found a fair-sized house that was once a Greek School and rejoices in the name of Pappadopol! Until we can find rooms we are to be quartered on the first floor. There are no drains, and we were decidedly peevish after viewing the premises. The rest of the unit and most of all the sanitary inspector even more so. Our belongings were brought down in ox-waggons. Twelve in our room—orderlies I mean, not ox-waggons.

December 24th. Galatz.

Having developed a violent toothache I slept badly, and am as cross as the tongs. We begin work in hospital tomorrow. Sister C. is suspected of diphtheria.

I orderlied for Dr. I., and asked to stay on for another six months. M. is the only other orderly who is staying in A. Camp. The guns in the Dobrudja direction very clear all day. No one seems to know for certain whether or not Tultcha has fallen, but rumour has it that our transport are back at Reni. Tultcha is important in that it commands one of the branches of the Danube delta, and, in consequence, an access to the Black Sea.

December 25th (Christmas Day). Galatz.

No work to be done except for the *sanitars*, who were kept busy stuffing mattresses. Everyone was rather too obviously cheerful, and I spent the afternoon with the dentist and made my toothache far worse.

They have flung a pontoon bridge across the Danube here, and the Dobrudja guns sound nearer.

A mail came in, but there was not one letter for any of us—all for Hospital B. and the transport! It was bitter.

A most wonderful spread awaited us at tea, and we played games and chanted carols far into the night. I'm sure the Russkis think we worship strange gods indeed!

To bed on 30 grains of Aspirin and two Somnytics, I should imagine a record.

December 26th. Galatz.

We were woken at 2 a.m. by a terrific explosion, followed by two less violent. It proved to be a Zeppelin—our first night raid—and the bombs were very near. The dentist later, but he did no good. News is bad and plans uncertain. Tultcha fell last Thursday or Friday, and our transport are believed to be at Ismail.

December 27th. Galatz.

Everyone busy getting the mattresses made and stuffed. I had a large tooth removed and am thankful.

Iliatchenko, the chief of the Russian Red Cross in these parts, visited the hospital. He said that in four or five days they will know whether or not it is possible to hold the line from a point between Issacea and Macin in the Dobrudja, up to Buzei, where a battle is now raging. If Macin falls Galatz must follow in three or four days' time, in which case we are to move north to Folteste, which lies at the head of a pontoon bridge on the Pruth, and set to work there. The transport have done very good work in the Dobrudja.

Commander Locker Lampson's armoured cars have all turned up here. They say Galatz will be bombarded from two sides, and blown to little, little bits. Today the guns were incessant.

We moved into our billets. M., N., S., B., and I are all together in a wee cottage 50 yards from the hospital.

December 28th. Galatz.

I am to have a ward to myself, and am absolutely *thrilled*. The second upstairs ward is nearly finished, but mercifully there are no wounded yet, and we ought to be quite ready by tomorrow. There is a rumour of a Russian victory.

December 29th. Galatz.

At work until 6 p.m., getting the three top wards ready. They look very nice, particularly my own!

I escaped for an interval after luncheon, and had a big wash in a small, small basin. A wonderful day, but no news, and only some letters for Hospital B. and the transport.

CHAPTER 5

January

December 30th—January 7th, 1917. Galatz—Reni.

I have had no time in which to write since the 30th. It has been a pretty terrible week, and one which not one of us is likely to forget.

On the afternoon of the 30th we admitted 100 wounded, on the evening of the 1st 160, and we evacuated from Galatz in the early hours of the 5th.

The school being originally for both boys and girls, was divided into two parts. We knocked a hole in the wall of partition, and by means of a precipitous ladder-like erection allowed the two to communicate. And here a word of sympathy for our poor old *sanitars* (Russian orderlies), who toiled gallantly up and down with the heavy stretchers all the day and most of the night. On the ground floor was the dressing-room, the wash-house, and two wards; on the first, three wards, the theatre, and the staff's united kitchen-mess room.

Dr. I. met every case at the door; when they wanted immediate attention they were sent straight to the two other doctors in the dressing-room, and the rest came to the wash-house. Later the rush was too great, and we had to give up the idea of undressing and washing every patient, though the joy the lighter cases took in their tubs of water was pathetic to behold. We worked by the inadequate illumination of a few oil lamps, and here and there a candle. It all seemed dim and confused. The whole of the first night I worked in the bath-room, and the uniform orderly had her work cut out indeed collecting the rags and scraps of uniforms into ordered bundles and seeing to their disinfection.

It is no light job undressing and washing a badly wounded six-foot-odd Russian who cannot understand what you want of him. When they realise we are English, they are nearly always confident

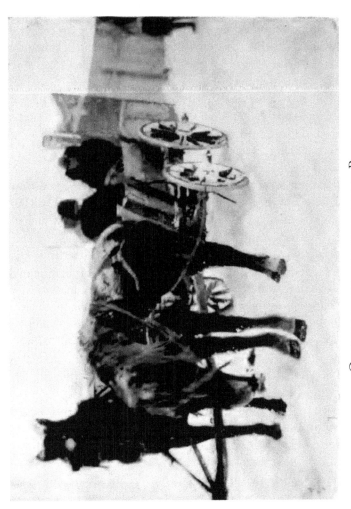

OFF ON A FORAGING EXPEDITION AT RENI

and friendly. And all the time the lamp flutters, and smokes, and smells, and as often as not in the end goes out.

We try and keep some record of each case; the name, number, and regiment, and we tie little cardboard discs round their necks with duplicate information. But so many come in dying or unconscious or delirious, and if they die I suppose no one ever discovers who or what they are or where they come from. And I suppose their families just go on—waiting. It makes one long wildly for law and order and discipline, whatever the picturesque value of other qualities. When these poor broken creatures are brought here in the springless carts to find, at the best, a straw mattress to lie on, to have to suffer tortures which perhaps they don't understand, with all day the horror of gangrene or tetanus before their eyes, and all day and all night long the smell, the confusion and the dirt—I think it is hard to realise until you have seen it the heartbreaking courage and loneliness of them all.

Some of them mere children, submitting quite quietly to a crippling operation; others peevish and indignant, imploring you to stop the pain; here and there a smile, and you don't know how we blessed the men who smiled; a child dying with a tiny abdominal wound; two delirious head cases; and in one corner an officer, blind and sullen, watched over by a devoted little Cossack servant. You thank Death whenever it comes, and often and often you pray that it may be quick, and every minute there is so much to do and every minute what you achieve must fall so short of the necessity. You don't know what it is to feel impotent like that.

It is no consolation to think that these men after all expect so much less than our own—they do no doubt—but that only makes it worse. They have led grey, grey lives always, and now they are dying this slow grey death.

We have only six trained sisters, and when you have taken off one for the theatre and two for night duty, three only are left for the wards. The other two nursing orderlies work in the theatre. At one time the sister and I on the first floor had over 90 patients between us. My ward was eventually just filled with straw, and the men were laid side by side as they came in as close as possible. We had an amazing percentage of very heavy cases, and were on every day, without a stop, up to anything between 2 and 6 the following morning. In the first 38 hours the doctors operated for 36 on end. The B.A.C. (British Armoured Cars) surgeon, Mr. Scott, came up to help, and brought with him four English orderlies who proved the most unutterable blessing.

On the afternoon of the 4th we got orders to evacuate at once, and immediately after Mr. Scott arrived and insisted that we should go to Reni on the A.C. barge that evening. Every patient that could be moved we sent off, and four of the unit stayed behind, with Dr. I. to look after those who could not go until the next day or were dying. The rest of us, which of course includes Sambo, got into the barge at 2 a.m. It was wonderful having everything smoothly and expeditiously arranged for us by English Tommies.

Galatz has been a nightmare, and I could not be sorry to go if it were not that we were once more retreating.

It was a beautiful night on the quay, with a burning granary making a terrific conflagration on the other side of the river, and the guns very near. They say Galatz will be shelled soon, and we heard—but this was only rumour—that Braila had fallen.

The hold was prepared for us, and we spent a comfortable night, and were woken up next morning by a cheerful Tommy with a bowl of steaming porridge. We did not leave Galatz until 8.30 a.m., and the journey to Reni took 1½ hours. A perfect day, and we have been given a nice little house here. We moved our stuff and ourselves, and the other four arrived next morning. Our orders point to our being sent to Kagul, north of Reni, and away from the railway, but this awaits official confirmation. It is very cold and there is some snow. The transport have all gone back to Odessa, as their cars have got to be repaired.

January 8th. Reni.

The news about Braila is true.

Damp, mud knee deep, and no news. The A.C. sent us two days' rations.

January 9th. Reni.

The six monthers left, travelling to Odessa on the A.C. train. B. is doing the kitchen, with me as her assistant!

One of the A.C. officers sent the "Scottish lasses" a truly wonderful present of butterscotch and peppermint creams. They are good to us.

January 10th. Reni.

After breakfast B. and I went on a foraging expedition. We got an order for meat from the *intendant de ville*, and the butcher was charming; but it was three hours before that meat arrived! In the end we returned to the Unit in triumph with half an ox, and a gorgeous supply of apples and onions.

The guns from Galatz thundered all day.

After supper I tried to cope single-handed with the porridge. L. came to the rescue, and saved the situation and the porridge just in time, but we both had to sit up until 11 stirring.

It is all hideously depressing: Galatz. No news. No mail. The party that has gone home. Retreats, and *mud*.

January 11th. Reni.

Mrs. H. and a mail arrived from Odessa soon after breakfast. No papers and no parcels, but lots and lots of letters. We spent a great morning reading, even though they seem pretty depressed at home, and to improve matters still more the sun came out and dried up some of the mud and my porridge wasn't so bad after all!

After tea a Russian officer in command of a battery here took us up to see it. Immensely interesting, dug-outs, trenches, wire entanglements, and field telephone all complete. The battery goes into action tomorrow.

We hated Reni that day we first saw it all hot and dusty last August. But the country behind is really full of possibilities, and you get a wonderful view of the grey river and the Dobrudja mountains.

A Bulgar shell burst in the river this afternoon, and Galatz was very busy and noisy. The remaining A.C. officers arrived from there, and came to supper, which they declared was good, although B. and I were not feeling at all equal to the occasion. They gave us some food, including a whole live sheep.

C. has gone home. The transport have broken up, and the cars will be useless until the spring.

Iliatchenko has been superceded, and our new chief, Prince Kropenski, is said to be coming here tomorrow.

January 12th. Reni.

Prince Kropenski arrived soon after breakfast; he speaks English perfectly, and has even played golf at St. Andrews! We are to stay here for the moment, and if the place is bombarded move to Bender. He has given us part of the barracks as a hospital, and a house near by to live in. We move at 8 a.m. tomorrow.

Kitchen and the toothache all day—heartily sick of both.

January 13th. Reni.

We have the most adorable house to live in that someone must have invented for a joke. It stands high, about a quarter of a mile back from the river, with a very fine view of the Danube and Galatz, over

68

which the shells are bursting. The hospital is to be in the barracks just below, and we spent the whole day getting the equipment up. M. has found a deserted black kitten, and so is, of course, perfectly happy! N. and I were left alone to cope with the dinner, which was a great success. They have sent for two more sisters from Hospital B. at Odessa, as well as cooks.

I do hope we shall get a chance of staying here.

January 14th. Reni.

It was moonlight when I got up this morning, and I got the breakfast by the help of the sunrise. The sunshine continues, and we live in our overalls; it's delicious.

Austrian prisoners are to work for us as *sanitars* in the hospital, and every drop of water we use for drinking and for the hospital has to be carted up from the river. And such water! It's the same colour as the tea, only it is opaque instead of clear. And by now we know our Danube too well to really enjoy drinking it. Soup made with it looks lovely so rich and thick.

January 15th. Reni.

Patients were promised to us by 12 a.m., but the hospital in the village was evacuated, and no train has come in yet. The wards look very nice, and we have actually got beds. Just plain wooden erections, little more than planks on a stand, but ever such a luxury for all that. I am in charge of the two straw wards.

The Russian evacuation hospital at the station is by way of sending us the bad cases that cannot travel any farther, and in the village there is a fever hospital for cholera and typhus. The prisoners are nice, and after the Russkis amazingly quick and clean.

A battery that lives about 300 yards away suddenly went off during luncheon, and made the most appalling noise.

January 16th. Reni.

The wounded started coming in at 1 a.m., but the night sisters managed nobly, and we were not had out of bed. Fifty admitted in all, and twenty more during the day. The cases are, on an average, better than at Galatz. On up till 9.30 p.m.

There appeared to be a great fire at Galatz, somewhere near the region of Pappadopol, and the bombardment was incessant. Here there was an aeroplane raid, which we and the Austrians watched side by side with equal interest.

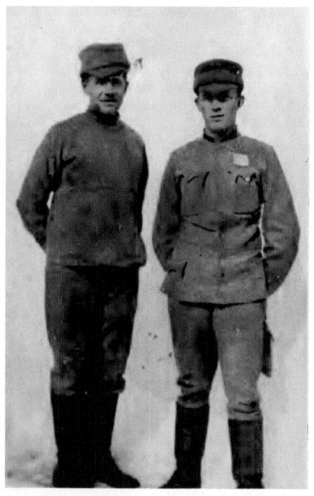

"LLSHKA AND BENDER, OUR AUSTRIAN COOKS."

January 17th. Reni.

Sambo has received official recognition. It became necessary. Dogs and puppies abound, and the Unit is developing a weakness for the adoption of any and every waif they meet. So now we have: "The Official Dog." Dr. I. loves him, as we all do, and even poor unofficial Pushkin (the black kitten) has almost won her heart.

Wards all day up to 12 p.m. No news, and the firing less violent.

January 18th. Reni.

We hear there is still some hope of holding Galatz and that Reni is a very strong position, so we look like staying here. Today Scotch mist and rain, with the wood supply threatening to give out. Most of our Austrians have been to Siberia, and now imagine themselves to be in a sort of paradise—poor devils.

January 19th. Reni.

Wards all day. We are getting much straighter, and it is a comfort not to be working in a blind chaos. I feel we have got the chance of doing real good to this lot, and the little Russian beds make such a difference. Tonight a snow blizzard.

(*Extract from a letter.*)

There were just two very characteristic sayings in Rumania. The first was: "*A la guerre comme à la guerre,*" applicable to every discomfort from a retreat to an attack of "cold feet," and the other: "*Les Alliés feront quelquechose.*"

I think I will bring back two Russkis together with their wives and families, and I gather the latter are extensive, to live at the lodge at Frogmore. Feodor is very good-looking, and David has a round red face like a gnome and cherishes an enormous beard. But I think they would both look picturesque in Camberley!

Rumour says that one method of censoring here is to delay all letters for four weeks without opening them, so that any information they might contain would be useless.

One of the cooks has just arrived from Odessa with a perfectly wonderful mail including parcels. Oh, such fun as it was—and I got a book besides a balaclava, a woolly cap, two pairs of woolly gloves, a housewife and three handkerchiefs. The winter has come at last too, so they have arrived just at the right moment.

You should have seen the mess-room last night. Supper cooled itself wearily on the table, while the entire unit sat buried in papers, letters, and parcels. The floor was soon invisible beneath a pile of paper, etc. Everyone presents a strangely bulgy appearance for days after a mail, as we have to go on duty with as much of it as possible stuffed into our pockets!

Our kit-bags are all in Odessa, and we left Braila on December 6th, anticipating a separation of, at the most, ten days! You all sound more cheerful, which is comforting—and have even mentioned peace terms. Does one? Is it the right thing to do in the best circles? How wonderful.

The cold weather is rather marvellous, and came quite suddenly after five glorious days of spring and sunshine. Now the ice is thick, thick, on our windows—you can see nothing at all of the outside world. The snow has already drifted very deep in places, and there is a bitter north wind blowing across the *steppe*.

January 20th. Reni.
This morning a telegram ordering instant evacuation caused the uttermost consternation, but was mercifully contradicted later. An awful day, snow drifting feet deep, bitterly cold and a wild blizzard. F. arrived in the evening from Odessa with letters.

Captain B., a Russian officer, has been sent to us by headquarters at Bolgrad in the place of the Russian sister, and to act as administrator and interpreter. He speaks English with a fearful stammer, and is quite diverting. My first meeting with him was in the ward. He came up to me and very gravely announced that one of the patients was suffering from "d-d-d-dreadful h-h-h-hills o-of the sh-shshtomack!"

January 22nd. Reni.
Heavy day, three cases in my ward desperately ill. Dr. I. went off to Odessa on business.

January 23rd. Reni.
Work much lighter. The local priest, the biggest man I have ever, ever seen, came to luncheon. He made the food look so inadequate that I felt quite sorry for it!

January 25th. Reni.
Twelve admitted. A busy day, but off after tea.

January 27th. Reni.
Busy day, a rumour about that Braila has been retaken, and fried eggs on toast for supper! The line between here and Galatz is under fire, which explains why our convoys always arrive at night.

L. is at this moment making a hideous noise, endeavouring to kill a centipede. It sounds easy, but the centipedes here are hard and scaly and quite four inches long. They scrunch—horrible! I wonder if St. George's dragon scrunched?

January 28th. Reni.

Snowing very hard. A little paralysed boy in my ward died—I am glad, poor child.

Prince O., the chief of the Red Cross in the whole of Russia, and a gentleman of quite dizzy eminence, was to have visited us today, but he never arrived.

(Extract from a letter.)

B. is making the pudding for supper and chanting in a doleful voice:

"The jam has given out,

"The marmalade has given out,

"The butter has given out,

"The margarine has given out."

The sad voice of an invalid is heard to murmur:

"And what *are* we going to eat?"

B. *(sternly)* "Bread and rice."

Outside the country is just a white glare, and floweth not with milk and honey; inside we can see very little, except the wonderful patterns the frost has made on our windows.

The other day we had a visit from some Russian military big-wig, who inspected the hospital. He examined everything in the most portentous silence, and we began to get nervous. Then—

"At last," he said—"at last I see women work." And the compliment to us, if not to our sex, was not a bad one.

I like the snow sometimes. It stops the guns, and makes the world a more peaceful place. Today there has been a heavy fall. To cheer us we hear there is better news. Wouldn't it be thrilling if our next move were an advance!

January 29th. Reni.

In bed all day with a bad pain and rather sick. Mrs. H. turned up late. She has been at Galatz all this time visiting the Front. The Braila rumour is untrue, but nevertheless the situation is quite encouraging. The line is held on the Sereth, and they say that all the German troops have been withdrawn from this Front.

Some of our men were evacuated today. They go in the same open carts even in this awful weather. It's an appalling thought. They would hardly be given so much as straw and blankets if we did not send our own.

It may be worth while to mention here that on one occasion during the worst of this terrible weather one of the aforementioned carts arrived, and when we went to carry the wounded in we found only two bodies frozen stiff under coverings that were just a sheet of ice. They had only about a quarter of a mile to travel to reach us. This may serve as an example of the conditions under which the men fight over here, with no hope of a Commission of Enquiry.

January 30th. Reni.
Off. Bitterly cold.

January 31st. Reni.
Off. A frightful blizzard, and collapse of the wood and water supply. The problem seems to be getting serious. We melt snow to meet the latter demand, and it certainly looks a more healthy drink than the Danube. We use it in hospital too. And instead of wood we burn reeds. They don't give much heat, and they are very extravagant, but there is nothing else. Here the mess-room fire is the only one allowed, and that is lit in the afternoon and kept going until after dinner.

Colder than ever, with a bitter wind. I suffered a severe relapse, and had to stay in bed, toothache being added to my other woes. I read *Ouida* all the morning and worse rubbish, if possible, all the afternoon. Like the melted snow and the reeds there is nothing else.

CHAPTER 6

February

February 2nd. Reni.

Off. Floods of sunshine, and I went down to the river. It was grey and unfriendly, with great blocks of ice floating along. The snow is blinding. We decorated the walls with shadow profiles of ourselves, and in consequence have fewer illusions left than ever.

February 3rd. Reni.

Back on duty. The men were very nice, and the work as usual. There was a boy with a terrible wound in his thigh, from shrapnel, and he was getting on so well. Then yesterday he died—oh, it is hateful.

February 5th. Reni.

Forty-four admissions last night, but light cases for the most part. The Bulgars are only six kilometres from the farther bank of the Danube, and here we are between the first and second Russian lines of defence. What fun for us when they start bombarding! A hostile aeroplane was over today.

February 6th. Reni.

A busy day, and not quite so cold. The authorities sent us twenty horses from Bolgrad to do our carting, but nothing whatever to feed them on, and the poor brutes are now subsisting on the crusts of our black bread. Meanwhile bread, wood, and meat are all threatening total failure.

They say if it were not for the difficulty of Transport and the shortage of food we could sweep Rumania clear tomorrow. No news.

February 7th. Reni.

Our new doctor arrived from Odessa soon after breakfast, and brought a mail. Hospital B. has been ordered to the Bukovina Front.

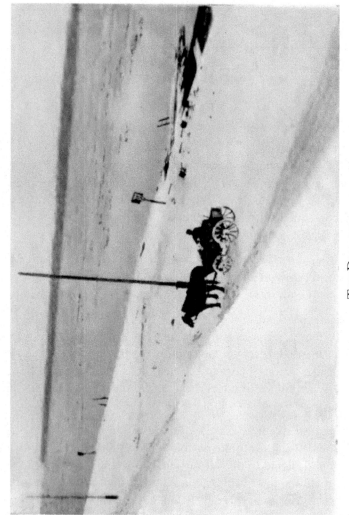

THE DANUBE

Dr. C. is to rejoin them, and so insisted on my coming to Odessa with her to get my teeth seen to.

Accordingly we embarked upon a sanitary (hospital) train at 8 p.m. Anyway the prospect of a kit-bag in the near future is alluring.

C. has joined the Anglo-Russian Hospital in Petrograd.

February 8th. In the Train.

We are travelling with something like 600 wounded. It is very comfortable. We share a carriage, have meals with the staff, and pay nothing. And such meals too. White bread and butter and *eggs*!

The train is in charge of a woman doctor, who speaks French, and is arranged as follows:

Coach No. 1 Isolation.
,, Nos. 2 and 3 Serious cases.
,, Nos. 4 and 5 Staff.
,, No. 6 Staff Dining-room and Office.
,, No. 7 Kitchen.
,, No. 8 *Sanitars'* quarters.
,, Nos. 9 and 10 Lighter cases.
,, No. 11 Dressing-room.
,, No. 12, etc. Wounded.

There was one German on the train, a prisoner, and very badly wounded. He looked so desolate that I felt surprisingly Christian all of a sudden, and even tried to talk German to him. He was being treated with every kindness and care. One cannot say too much for the way in which the first field dressings are done here, and every man has the date of his last dressing written on his bandages.

February 10th, Odessa.

We got into Odessa about midday, and two most delightful sleighs took us up to Hospital B. It's a truly magnificent place. Bathroom, electric light and radiators. The latest rumour says that Hospital B. is to go somewhere near Jassi, not to the Bukovina. Dr. I. has gone back to Reni.

February 14th. (Extract from a letter.)

I am having an excellent time here, and feel rather ashamed of myself, as you are probably picturing me being a noble woman under the worst possible conditions. The dentist is doing his lurid worst, and a toothless if painless future awaits me.

From you today two letters, some soup, a beautiful hanky and chocolate, of which the censor was good enough to leave me three bits!

We went for a picnic the other day. No one but the Scottish Women would have thought of it, I am certain. We sat in the snow, and drank tepid tea, and ate homemade dripping cake, with the bluest of Black Seas at our feet. It was great fun, and we laughed too often and too much to feel cold. Tonight one of the sisters has invited me to *Traviata*, and tomorrow I am going to *Prince Igor*, so I am lucky, for in Odessa we do things musical well.

February 15th. Odessa.

A glorious day. Up late and in the afternoon we went for a long sleigh drive, which was great fun, though far more nerve-racking than a retreat. The private sleighs are really beautiful, and great coloured nets are spread over the horses' backs and fly behind them as they move. The pavements are inches deep in ice, and walking is both difficult and perilous. Something like 30 degrees of frost to-day.

To tea and supper with a member of the English colony. Real English open fires and *buns!*

The docks are frozen hard, such a winter has been unknown for years.

February 18th. Odessa.

B. and N. arrived from Reni on their way back home. Life will be an utter blank without them. Mrs. M. is coming back with me.

February 20th. In the Train.

We left Odessa about 6 p.m. and have sixteen packages and cases of hospital stuff to steer safely to Reni. About 12 p.m. we got ourselves and our baggage into a sanitary train at Sastava, where a little Jew boy, with wavy golden hair and tight mauve mufti, made himself most agreeable in French.

February 21st. In the Train.

We saw a wolf quite close to the railway line, and so feel we have beheld true Russia at last! It is pathetic; they only give us one real meal a day, and we brought no provisions. Also I did think I was looking my very, very best in all the glories of a new uniform and Odessa-waved hair. But to no purpose. The mauve Jew became very confidential this morning, and gazing at my new, new tunic, said mournfully that it was sad indeed that we wore such clothes, for was it not the duty of every woman at least to *try* and look her best!

February 22nd. In the Train.

This morning the *sanitar* presented us with the bill for yesterday's food, together with a depressing breakfast of black bread and *tchi*. We stopped for 24 hours at Besserabski. No one was the least surprised—we do these things in Russia.

February 23rd. In the Train.

Started off again. An uneventful and rather hungry day.

February 24th. Reni.

Woke up at Reni, and by luncheon time had all our baggage safely unshipped.

There is a case of typhus in the hospital, so we are in quarantine for twelve days. On duty. Beds have been put in my ward, and it is opened whenever the others are over full.

We have a new Russian sister to help with the secretarial work; she looks a dear, and speaks English very well.

February 25th. Reni.

Work as usual. I miss B. and N. horribly.

CHAPTER 7

March

March 1st. Reni.

Wet, cold and horrible. No news.

March 2nd. Reni.

Today came the worst blizzard we have yet had. Almost cut off from the hospital. The Danube has been frozen hard for the last week, and is used as a means of communication with the opposite bank, which is guarded by Cossack patrols. Anyway, the carts are able to bring over some wood, which is something.

March 4th. Reni. (*Extract from a letter.*)

We have been gathering a little news of the outside world from a B.A.C. Officer, who has just come up from *tiraspol* (their base). The Russian commander-in-chief of this Front is by way of inspecting us this afternoon, and yesterday a big sanitary man came and held a bug hunt on a large scale.

But they all make pretty speeches, so I hope they are pleased.

March 7th. Reni.

Heavenly day—thawing. Work much as usual, and we evacuated twenty-nine men. I took rather a pleasant photograph of the sisters in their typhus kit. No news.

March 11th. Reni.

Cold and more snow. Kropenski arrived late, and expressed himself very pleased. Our little captain is to go, but the sister to stay.

March 12th. Reni.

Work as usual. I went for a long walk with M. We crossed the Pruth, and altogether covered about five miles. Got back after dark

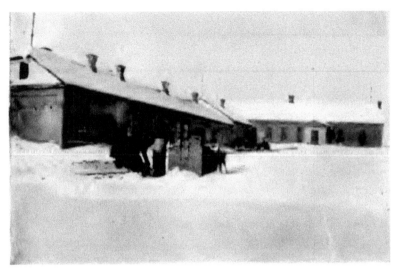

OUR HOSPITAL AT RENI.

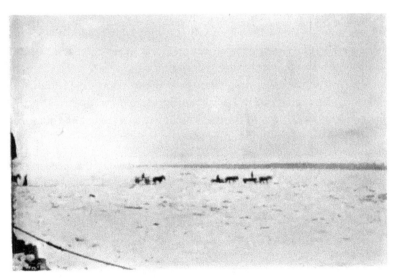

WOOD-CARTS CROSSING THE FROZEN DANUBE.

wading through seas of mud.

(*Extract from a letter.*)

This is bound to be a record of domestic happenings—the war being for the moment uneventful.

To begin at the very beginning, there is a convulsion of nature at 6.30 a.m., and an Austrian prisoner staggers in with two green canvas buckets full of water. Nice iced water! A few, and I am not of their number, wash. As Dr. I. says: "Some people will always wash, but others will only do so if it is made easy for them." Hence the buckets. Then we make our beds, and breakfast follows at 7.15. Room inspection at 5 to 8, and roll call at the hospital at 8. From 12 to 1.30 we alternately go to first and second dinner. If you go to first you come on immediately after until 5, and if to second you are off until 4.30. Tea is from 4 to 5, and supper from 7 to 8.15. After supper hot water is obtainable, and you will be relieved to hear that the family wash, unless the supply is low, in which case a hot water-bottle takes precedence. This is the routine, though it is often sadly mutilated by circumstances.

Mrs. M. feeds us wonderfully, and supplies are far more plentiful.

Last night I saw the most magnificent meteor.

A walk by the river is a curious sight these days. The bank is one long line of trenches and observation posts. Little houses are beginning to emerge above the snow, while others are still submerged, and the ice is on a level with the thatch. As soon as the ice breaks up the floods will be severe, and railway communication with Galatz will be cut off. You know, of course, that there is only one single line from here to Odessa, and a little light extension line on to Galatz. But that is the case in most parts of Russia, I believe. So, in these circumstances, you may imagine the difficulties of transport are immense, and more than ever so in this weather. The hardest winter they have had for nearly ten years.

I have just been down to see sixteen of our men off from the evacuation hospital—a striking contrast to seeing them off at Derby. The usual springless carts are sent for them; I got in with one of the stretcher cases, and off we bumped. (It's ghastly for the badly wounded.) I had on my Cossack hood, greatcoat, and high boots, and the driver was convulsed when he discovered I was not a soldier. He laughed, and I laughed, and the patients joined in—in fact, we thought it a very good joke indeed! I saw them into the train, and then started for home in one of the carts with my own *sanitar*. It is quite a short way, but the night is dark, and we managed to lose the track and get well stuck in the snow.

March 13th. Reni.

Very cold. Guns all day, and a part of Galatz seemed to be burning. The Russian batteries on our Right answered. The enemy shelled the Pruth defences, and one shell came over Reni, but did not burst.

Pushkin has eloped with an *enormous* grey tabby.

March 14th. Reni.

At supper we were sent a message: "Bagdad is by the English Army taken." Great news indeed, and the Russians are said to be drawing down from the north.

March 16th. Reni.

Wards slack. Captain B. departed in the evening. 'Th-ththank you s-s-s-so m-m-much for the b-b-b-beautiful k-kindness sh-shewn me in y-y-your middle,' was his farewell to the *Unit.*

March 17th. Reni.

Gorgeous day—went for a long walk. On the way to the Pruth watched a fine air-raid. All along large numbers of Austrian prisoners were digging trenches, etc., and the road was flooded in places. Beyond the Pruth the road was completely submerged, and the railway embankment was supplemented with sandbags. We walked until we were held up by water.

March 18th. Reni.

No one can think or speak of anything but the Revolution. Captain B. arrived post-haste from Bolgrad this morning to tell us the news, a gleam in his eye, and his stammer forgotten. The first tidings had come from the Turks in the Dobrudja, who had wirelessed their congratulations!

On February 26th (O.S.) the *Duma* had been dissolved, but had refused to disperse, and the abdication of the emperor was demanded. He obeyed, and they have now formed a provisional government. The throne was offered to the emperor's brother, Michail Alexandrovitch, but he will accept it only on condition that he is elected thereto by the entire nation. The Grand Duke Nicholas is once more in supreme command of the armies on all Fronts, and they say there will be a big move soon. There is the wildest enthusiasm and confidence everywhere, and they claim the whole Revolution to be the work of the army and people united. Splendid—*splendid.* The emperor is believed to be a prisoner at Tsarskoe.

Everyone is beaming, and one cannot even in these early days but rejoice at the change of attitude. One had heard and was weary of so much gossip.

We already talk of the *Ancien Régime!*

March 19th. Reni.

No news. The Danube is free. Pushkin returned to the family circle quite unrepentant.

March 20th. Reni. (*Extract from a letter.*)

We've had the most breathless and unexpected day. It began early this morning with the arrival of Kropenski, Prince Dolgoroukov, the commanding officer of the troops here, the commander-in-chief of the whole Front and all his gilded staff. After they had inspected the hospital, we were lined up in a row, and—decorated! We have got the "George," the same as the soldiers get, which adds to their value, and when we returned to the wards we created a far greater sensation than the Revolution ever did. I was very touched by the dear old N.C.O. of the Austrian prisoners, who saluted and congratulated me in German in the most delightful way.

(*From Diary.*)

An enemy aeroplane over and the shooting better. As a matter of fact, it is over at this minute. I am sitting out in brilliant sunshine, the batteries on either side of us have opened fire, and I can hear the shells buzzing through the air as I write.

March 22nd. Reni.

All leave is stopped on this Front. Work is slack, which Dr. I. says is bad for us, wherein I do not agree.

F. and I moved up to the turret, which is delicious.

March 23rd. Reni.

This morning the wards were blessed and *ikons* put up in each.

A Russian doctor visited the hospital in the afternoon, and shed some interesting light on the other side of the Revolution, *i.e.*, the democratic influence in the ranks. I should love to see them working out their own salvation, and in the end I am sure they will succeed; but the present possible effect of the Revolution on the army does undoubtedly make one anxious. They say the Socialistic element makes an unanimous election of the Grand Duke Michail Emperor impossible.

84

March 25th. Reni.

We have been making history by attending a Free Speech Revolutionary Meeting in the market square. The crowd was almost entirely composed of and addressed by soldiers and officers; the meeting was much beflagged in scarlet, and had a passion for singing the *Marseillaise*. But the gist of the speeches (as conveyed to us later by the Russian sister) was much to the point. They insisted that the first duty of the citizens of the Republic was to defend Russian soil, announced that proof of treasonable guilt on the part of the emperor and empress had been found, and added that whereas hitherto England and France had always doubted the good faith of Russia, henceforth her loyalty was assured, and the war would be fought to a finish. The audience was good-tempered and appreciative, and there came a charming interlude when they sang, as only Russians can sing, a little chant and prayer for all those killed at Petrograd during the Revolution.

Judging from this afternoon the only people in Russia who are not free-born are the people who disagree with you. They had a short way with hecklers!

Freedom of speech, letters, and religion is granted. So far so good. It is a big task for those responsible. The men are just beginning to realise the change, though to our eyes they seem slow to grasp it, and they are terribly dangerous material for the agitator.

One sees this even in hospital. The man with a little education has an enormous influence over the rest. And he is full of big, plausible ideas, as vague and as restless as his own discontent. And I don't think that the dullness of the average peasant is lethargy; on the contrary, they are inflammable and primitive. They reason like children, and are ignorant and affectionate like children—but they are also forceful and mysterious.

We have a very mixed lot in just now, and through our being in quarantine they have had to stay in some time, so that we have got to know them rather well.

For instance, in the ward in which I am working there is an unpleasant individual of "education" who talks a lot, and would no doubt give the Almighty advice on the creation of a new Heaven and a new Earth if he got the opportunity. Close to him an older man who looks like an Archangel, and argues gently all day, and in the corner behind the stove a sad misanthrope. But I like the latter, because he is intelligent, and though he may have come to much the same conclusions as my first friend he has suffered much on the way there.

There are many boys, dull and rather stupid, and then there is Simeon. Simeon is just the most beautiful male thing I have ever seen. I told the unit so, and they all flocked to look at him in bed with his cropped head, and they appreciated his manners and his beautiful smile, but went away disappointed. You are until you see him move. This utterly graceful creature is over six foot, is only nineteen and comes from Siberia. No, he says, he does not want to go home, he wants to go back to the Front, get another nice little wound and so return to the "*Schottlandski Lazaret*" (Scottish Hospital). And after a compliment like that, do you wonder that we all love him!

We have one "smart" young man, he can read and write, is a smith by trade, and in times of peace earns an astonishing number of *roubles* a month. If there is one thing he abhors it is the uneducated! And then there is Nikolai. Nikolai has been desperately ill and with us a long time. He will say you are the most perfect of created beings if he is feeling in the mood, and will bite you if he isn't. And so it goes on. The young ones are for the most part delightful, and young and old will, just like the Tommy at home, produce all his treasures to show you. Our youngest patient is a Cossack sergeant of fifteen. He was adopted by the regiment when a child, and has won all the four medals of St. George, and all the four crosses. He is quite frightfully naughty and a great darling.

As to the hospital, it is really very smart these days. It forms two sides of a square, and the men when they first come in are taken straight into the receiving-room, where they can repose on straw, and where they are given a hot bowl of *tchi* and some bread. Next door is the bathroom, and opening out of it the disinfecting-room, the uniform-room and the mortuary. We can house 150, and the wards, the store-room, and the theatre fill the rest of the building.

March 26th. Reni. (*Extract from a letter.*)
A very cold spell lately, but today again floods of sunshine.

We have seen the wild geese flying north, we have seen the storks beginning to nest, we have looted irises for our garden, and we have planted sunflowers. We are, in fact, happy and comfortable, and therefore expect to be forced to leave Reni before we are very much older! The hospital is fast filling up again.

The B.A.C.'s are in rather a pessimistic frame of mind.

Four of us have moved up to the turret, and yesterday I awoke to behold big fires on the slopes of the mountains opposite—signs of a

Bulgarian withdrawal that were confirmed later in the day. We hear, too, of a new German offensive with Petrograd as its objective, and of a French success at Verdun.

The roof collapses at short intervals, otherwise the turret is delicious.

Matron has gone off to Galatz to try and raise some firewood.

March 7th. Reni.

Yesterday an article in Polish appeared in one of the Russian newspapers, a remarkable sign of the times. The prisoners' N.C.O., who hails from Austrian Poland, nearly wept for joy, poor old dear.

Twenty slight cases admitted.

March 29th. Reni.

Matron back from Galatz and wood—we hope—to follow. She said Pappadopol still stands amidst the ruins of the Goods Station. The higher portions of the town have suffered very little.

I went for a long walk on the *steppe*, and found the "Happy Valley." In a week the whole place will be wonderfully alive. Back by the trenches and wire entanglements with a magnificent view of the whole country.

March 30th. Reni.

Endless operations. No news.

March 31st. Reni.

We evacuated thirty-five patients.

A number of troops left for the trenches at 6 a.m. At 8 the body of one soldier was brought back to our mortuary. He had shot himself this wonderful morning not more than a mile away.

I wonder if he had been there before—and knew, or if he had only sat and thought? His officer brought him back—a boy, very young and tense. The extraordinary beauty of the morning makes the tragedy, oh, so hopeless and unutterable. Everything seemed to say live—I wonder if the little soldier felt that too, or if he only heard the rumbling of the guns on the horizon.

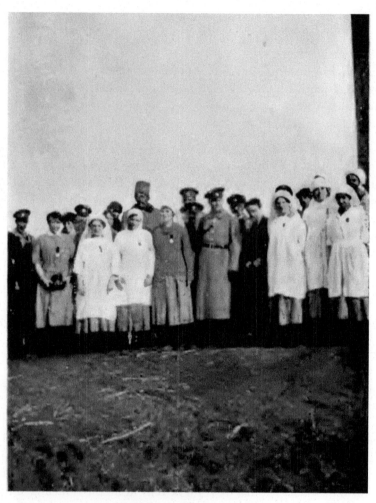

THE UNIT DECORATED.

CHAPTER 8

April

April 1st. Reni.

We admitted twenty-two. My ward opened for three query fevers. A heavenly day.

April 2nd. Reni

I went for a ride with M. after luncheon. It was great fun, but hard work from every point of view, for our steeds needed much encouragement. We found a new village possessed of two blue lakes and a wonderful view.

A successor to Captain B. has arrived—one Petrovitch. He speaks French, German, and Italian, was an opera singer, and is hampered by an artistic temperament, which he can never, never forget. He has a secretary too. A languid young man in a beautiful Cossack cloak—very long and curly (the cloak, I mean, not the young man).

April 5th. Reni.

A big bombardment as from beyond Galatz last night.

Our laundry superintendent's chiefest assistant has gone off to Galatz in company with a soldier. And poor dear T. was just contemplating taking her back to England to be the prop of her declining years! And that has not been her only disillusion of late. David—the laundry orderly—she loved very much, indeed so did we all. And he fell ill, which was very sad, for he was just about to go on leave; his wife had died, he did not know what might befall his daughters, and he had no news. We loaded him with sympathy, and then we made a fearful discovery—David was a Mohammedan, he had six wives, it was only the seventh who had died!

The B.A.C. Tommies apparently take quite a jealous interest in our welfare, and great rivalry exists in Odessa between them and the British Red Cross orderlies as to the superiority of either unit. And another story tells of a chilly Tommy on the quay at Galatz saying to his officer: "I hope you are not going to keep us here all night, Sir; remember we are not the Scottish Women!"

The weather is gorgeous, hot days and cool nights. The hospital is busy, though there has been no rush as yet, and the cases are light. Still, we have about fifty patients in, and receive and evacuate quite half that number every two or three days. We rather dread a move, for there would be little chance, I imagine, of doing more than retrace our footsteps for a month or two, and it would be awful to sit in Galatz or Braila all the summer. Of course, if we could sweep through Rumania, we would pack cheerfully tomorrow, but I suppose that is not to be expected.

There are great compensations to be had out of an uneventful existence here. We have started quite a large out-patients department for the troops of the Reni division, and the men flock in. They are most anxious to be received at the *"Angliscke Lazaret,"* and our reputation with them helps enormously in dealing with men from the Front. Now, they no longer look upon us as strangers, but arrive smiling, make friends, and are sorry to go. And we are often very sorry to lose them.

Riding is our newest diversion, and it is great fun. The steeds remind me chiefly of the seaside donkey of my youth, and the Cossack saddles cause us exquisite pangs; nevertheless, the horses are visibly improving, and I for one am not sorry they have lost something of their first fire!

April 7th. Reni. *(Extract from a letter.)*

A delirious, a positively delirious mail this morning. To make matters perfect F. got a day off for us both out of the authorities, so that it came about that the mail surprised us, having scrambled eggs for breakfast in the turret, where we proceeded to spend a blissful morning. Now, she and I and M. are away in that dip of the steppe, which we have christened the "Happy Valley," with luncheon, tea, and supper in our haversacks. The Happy Valley is cultivated here and there, and full of little fruit trees not yet in blossom, and of little queer flowers that are. There is a vineyard farther up, and a stream down the middle, with big, big walnut-trees alongside. And everywhere flocks of sheep, and altogether delightful shepherd babies.

Later.

We did about 10 miles after I wrote this yesterday. Our new village was too fascinating for anything. There were the blue lakes and the willows, very soft and grey and young, and large black and white storks balancing themselves in pools—all for us!

April 8th. Reni.

America has declared war on Germany.

April 9th. Reni.

Kropenski's son came to supper very lugubrious about the Revolution, and there are sinister rumours of wholesale mutiny and desertion from Galatz. Reni was bombarded, and the situation is obviously critical.

April 10th. Reni.

The fever hospitals at Galatz are reported full of typhus, but very few wounded are coming in. Braila is still an island, and the snow from the Carpathians has yet to thaw, which will flood the place again.

April 13th. Reni.

After tea I proposed a walk to M. and we started for the Happy Valley. All the cherry blossom was in flower and innumerable beasts and green things flourished.

April 15th (Easter Day, O.S.). Reni. (*Extract from a letter.*)

We are enjoying our Russian Easter. I have just been down to the wards. They were full of sailors up from the quay laden with bowls of white bread, coloured eggs, Easter cake, and bottles of wine, of all of which we were made to partake. And too I like the greeting:

Christos Voskrese!" (Christ is risen.)

—and the answer: *Voistenoo Voskrese.* (He is risen indeed.)

After luncheon the *sanitars* all trooped up to the house to receive their Easter present of money. First they tossed the doctors, and then they cheered all those who have fallen in the war, and the English sisters. We in our turn cheered Russia. During the afternoon there was another outburst of cheering and Colonel —— was carried to the door of the hospital by his men. He made a tour of the wards with his staff, greeting and kissing every man in turn. After tea the *sanitars* gave an entertainment in the courtyard of the hospital, and we saw some really beautiful dancing. F. and I. danced the polka with them, and later performed the Highland Schottische with immense success! A sailor played the *balalaika* and sang—a really enchanting performance.

There are sundry gloomy rumours about chief amongst them that of a Russian evacuation of Galatz.

April 16th. Reni.

The Galatz news is untrue, and a big English success in France is reported in the papers.

The sailors gave an entertainment this evening in the ward, singing to the accompaniment of a guitar and a *balalaika*. The men sit enthralled, and the music is often beautiful.

The colonel came up to supper. In Russia, at least, Easter is a real festival.

All the Austrian prisoners who have, up till now, been quartered in the Pruth village are to be moved back; two Russian regiments are to take their place.

April 17th. Reni.

A wild storm from midday on, hailstones quite an inch in diameter, and all the windows on the weather side of the hospital are broken. Had a half day.

April 18th. Reni.

Work uneventful, but the turret spent a ridiculous night. The ceiling, which is made of mud, fell about us in chunks, owing to a leaking roof and much rain. It was impossible to deal with the situation, so we buried ourselves under ground sheets and mackintoshes, took our valuables to bed with us, and hoped for the best!

April 19th. Reni.

I am told this weather lasts a fortnight—will the turret? This morning our floor was a sea of liquid mud; here and there a sort of bog stopped all progress, and gumboots were the only possible form of bedroom slipper. Soon we shall give way altogether, and collapse on to the heads of the sisters below.

The Bulgarian guns that had been bombarding Reni have been silenced by our own. But they are now mounting a 12-inch gun out of range of ours, and capable of knocking us to bits. A gas attack is also threatened.

Two nice A.C. Tommies came in to supper, and there is a vaguely hopeful air about the rumours.

April 20th. Reni.

Fine but chilly. A new patient developed typhus.

April 21st. Reni.

Two A.C. Tommies spent the day here on their way through from Galatz to Tiraspol. They said that the literature dropped in the Russian trenches by the Bulgarians at Easter was full of the abuse of England, and very cleverly written. They only made one mistake. They said we were responsible for the deposition of the Romanoffs.[1]

April 22nd—26th. Reni.

Nothing of importance, changeable weather, air-raids. A sinister rumour about that Russia means to make a separate peace, but we refuse to believe it.

I rode this evening with M. A good little horse, and it was great fun.

Our Austrian orderlies have been taken away, and replaced by a new lot—much weeping and gnashing of teeth.

April 27th. Reni.

Cold. Air-raids. Work as usual.

April 28th. Reni.

M., F., and I moved into tents. We were given one apiece—heavenly.

April 29th. Reni.

Rode with Sister G. The men were evacuated.

April 30th. Reni.

This morning an enemy aeroplane was brought down behind the Bulgarian lines by a Russian machine.

(Extract from a letter.)

I have got one entire tent to myself. I wonder if you can realise what that means after a minimum of four in a room? I moved yesterday, and in consequence my temper is becoming momentarily more angelic. To wake up in the morning and find yourself lord of a kingdom 8 x 10 is real bliss. The weather is uncertain, and prone to violent storms of wind and rain—I hope the kingdom won't collapse! The art of keeping warm *in* bed I have brought to perfection.

One of the patients was heard to remark the other day: "The Rus-

---

1. *The Last Days of the Romanovs* by George Gustav Telberg & Robert Wilton - The Murder of the Tsar & the Russian Royal Family, 1918 is also published by Leonaur.

sian sisters are pretty, but they are not good—the English sisters are good, but they are not pretty!" We are very cast down.

Dr. I. is getting very restless, the fighting on this Front seems so long delayed, and believes that the Serb division will soon want us again, though whether for work here or to follow them to Salonica seems uncertain. Of news from Petrograd we have none.

The birds in the Happy Valley are thrilling us. There are bright blue birds and golden birds, there are horsey-looking fellows in black and white check—magpies galore—hawks, buzzards, storks, and cocky-oily birds of all sorts, sizes, and tongues.

We have only 40 patients in, but as the cases now are mostly medical or else sent in for operation a good deal of the work is interesting and new.

CHAPTER 9

May

May 1st. Reni.

We sang the *Marseillaise,* and waved blood-red banners all day. It is a good safety valve, I suppose, if not exactly business. I rode with Dr. I., and went for a walk with M. after supper. A gorgeous night.

May 2nd. Reni.

One bit of good news today. The Turks and the Bulgarians are fighting amongst each other in the Dobrudja. It's more than we do anyway—fighting.

Galatz was heavily shelled. A poor little lunatic boy was brought in this evening by his N.C.O. He would insist on taking his trousers off, and dictating peace terms to the *Kaiser* through the lamp wires.

I had a day off, and a long walk with M.

May 3rd. Reni.

No news, wet and windy.

May 5th. Reni.

Matron was stopped by some soldiers on her way into the village this morning, who asked her if we had everything we wanted—for if not, *they* would see that we got it! And Nikolai distinguished himself by telling four Russian doctors who were paying us a state visit that no Russian hospital he'd ever seen was anything like as good as ours!

Air-raids.

I went for a long picnic walk with M. and F. First we dawdled down the Happy Valley, and the valley that is beyond. This brought us to a big farm, all orange in the sunset, and after we had successfully surmounted the usual obstacles in the form of the decaying corpses of horses and cattle, we found a golden green field" where we ate our

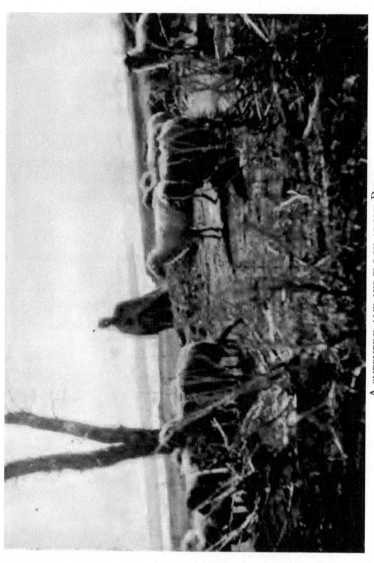

A SHEPHERD AND HIS FLOCK ABOVE RENI

supper. By then the sun had disappeared and the world grown chilly, so we struck out through a belt of trees and made for high open ground. When we reached the Pruth, well above the village, we sat down to rest. The moon had not yet risen, and in the brown shadow of the twilight we watched the red glow die over Galatz.

And then we said we'd go home. We did not dare make for the familiar shore road, as we were behind the defences, and would probably have been shot at sight, so we kept inland—and walked. We got completely lost, and when we found a landmark we were quite 5 miles the farther and the wrong side of Reni. But it was well worth it. There was a wonderful moon, and we seemed all alone in an utterly soundless world. Wherever we looked, the sweep of plain, and now and then the gleam of the river in the distance.

May 6th. Reni.

Work as usual. The troops had a field day, or rather a field night, and rushed yelling round our tents for hours.

May 8th. Reni.

Miss H. and an enormous mail arrived about 10 p.m., but my news was not good.

May 9th. Reni.

We were heavily bombarded this afternoon, and a shell burst only 100 yards from the hospital. It was interesting to watch. The Bulgars had sighted our nearest battery. We could see the puff of their guns as they were fired and the shells bursting this side, and we could watch our return fire equally well.

May 10th. Reni.

A smallpox out-patient. Huge excitement and much waving of Typhol.

It is decided that I ought to go home, though it's very, very hard to leave. Simeon was delightful, and Sister G. gave a lovely farewell supper-party for me. We sang songs, and watched the most amazing summer lightning playing over Galatz.

May 11th. Reni.

Wet and wild. I went to the Happy Valley. It was very grey and sad.

May 12th. In the Train.

Left Reni. *Miserable.*

May 14th. Odessa.

I had a somewhat verminous journey here, sandwiched in between free-born Russians. We were kicked out at Odessa at 4 a.m. this morning. I went to the waiting-room, until N. turned up about 6, and had a long conversation with a really interesting Russian. He was a Socialist, who had before the war travelled all over Europe studying economic conditions.

N. took me to a very welcome bath, bed, and breakfast. The state of things here is a revelation. They are on the eve of a pogrom, the Jew element is synonymous with the German, and their organisation for propaganda marvellous. Only this evening a telegram was published in the papers announcing that the Allies had demanded the instant suppression of the Soviet (Soldiers' and Workmen's Committees). The telegram was traced to a Jewish source—denied, and the edition as far as possible confiscated—but the harm was done. Every minute makes leaving harder.

In the evening the consul telephoned to say I could catch the train for Petrograd tomorrow morning at 7.

May 18th. Petrograd.

I reached Petrograd this morning. The train was very crowded, and we travelled by the most direct and the dullest route, touching neither Kiev nor Moscow. I met one interesting man, the head of the Food Supply Department for Odessa City. He spoke perfect English, and in spite of the alarming price of food in Odessa—supplies being largely in the hands of the Jews—was not unduly pessimistic. Nevertheless, the food problem is responsible for much that is critical in the present state of unrest.

There were some abominable Jews in the next-door carriage, who pretended they were English, and tried to scrape acquaintance the whole way. The North does not in an equal degree share the feeling of South Russia against the race, so doubtless this party consider that for the moment the North is a healthier place of residence. In my own carriage a most unpleasant Russian lady, but it all might have been a great deal worse.

I drove straight to Mrs. L.'s house from the station, and found to my dismay that she had left for Christiania the day before. The hotels I knew were all overflowing, and I was in the middle of pondering my next move, when a youthful Englishman appeared from nowhere in particular and offered me a telephone and two bachelor flats. I accepted the first, and telephoned to C. at the Anglo-Russian hospital. She was in, so I climbed back into my *isvostchik* and drove there. The hospital is in the Dmitri Palace on the Nevski, a huge and wonderful place. The matron invited me to lodge at their nurses' home—a reincarnated night club—so C. and I went off there together. In the afternoon I imbibed new sights, sounds, and smells, and left a note at the embassy. The streets are full of soldiers, but quite quiet, and the crowd on the Nevski makes progression infinitely slow.

The population, thanks to Polish refugees and the enforced residence of most of the richer people, is now 3,000,000 as against 1,000,000 in time of peace. There are no police, trams are so crowded there is not even toe-room, *isvostchiks* are as ruinous as they are dishonest and the distances are enormous. I saw *real* gipsies for the first time—none of your weary, dreary, poaching English variety, but ladies with a sense of colour and a very distinct sense of the dramatic. Mongolians, too, with century-old padded coats, very beautiful as to colour, but—unclean.

Beggars innumerable and picturesque, but also—a sordid disgrace—mutilated soldiers begging in the streets under a government begging licence. Lepers, of course, for on the outbreak of the Revolution these too declared themselves free-born, and are now enjoying the fruits of liberty with the rest of the citizens of this millennium. Which reminds me of a story I heard in Odessa. When the prisoners there were released the first thing they did was to elect the chiefest criminal amongst them governor of the gaol.

The victims of the Revolution are buried—inadequately—in the Champ de Mars. At first it was the people's wish that the spot chosen should be the gardens of the Winter Palace; this was over-ruled, but I like it—the suggestion that these martyrs should lie forever in the House of the Romanoffs.

The Champ de Mars is railed off in the centre and makes a convenient rallying ground for the discontented, from soldiers to schoolchildren.

May 19th. Petrograd.

Had luncheon at the embassy, and in the evening they telephoned asking me to come and stay.

May 20th. Petrograd.

To the embassy at tea-time. I landed in the middle of a tea-party, and wished I didn't look so like an eccentric boy scout.

May 21st. Petrograd.

I have got the most heavenly room looking out on the Neva, with the most heavenly bed where breakfast finds me in the morning, and is followed by a yet more heavenly bath next door. The difficulties of getting out of the country are enormous, and I chase my passport all day.

May 31st. In the Train. Petrograd–Torneo.

C. and I left Petrograd this morning. It has been a wonderful time, and I want to go back worse than ever.

To begin with, it is a really beautiful city, though it is built on a marsh, and the climate is vile. I arrived in a snowstorm, and today it is almost too hot to breathe. And always, always, a hot and dusty wind, or a cold and snowy one. But there are compensations. I don't wish for anything much more satisfactory than to be out about 2 a.m. in a clear blue twilight, with sunset and sunrise getting entangled across the river. Or more beautiful than, say, the spire of the fortress of Peter and Paul, the colour of the blue Mosque opposite, or the huge Palace of Metchnikoff—Peter the Great's friend.

The churches are disappointing, but I like the instinct that enclosed the gutter, the rail, and the pavement on which the body of Alexander II. fell within the church raised on the spot to his memory. That dusty bit of road is a better monument than most.

It is significant that now the churches are deserted, for if ever a people possessed an instinct for religion, a profound "will" for it, the Russian does. And one realises, too, that Petrograd is modern in the wide sense; it is the centre only in name. Here come most elements from the outside world, and fewest from real Russia. Everything that is disloyal, everything that is feverish and uncertain, the soldier who wants peace and plenty without further trouble, a tragically childish outlook on the part of the ignorant population—in itself a confession of what they have suffered—or else a tragically superficial one from the man who cannot read or write, but is told he is henceforward the ruler of his country.

But through it all you find expressed suddenly and unerringly an amazingly direct instinct for what is beautiful—in the city, in colour here, in music there, in books, in painting, in the theatre, in a peasant's choice of an expression. It is the stamp of an individuality, and it breaks through at moments when indolence and corruption seem to have won the day and surely with a promise for the future.

Meanwhile it is not a little humorous to walk past the figure of the autocratic Catherine on the Nevski, for she holds in her hand today a small and very modern red flag! Not far away is the Astoria Hotel, which suffered so much at the hands of the Revolutionary troops. One of their own generals had given his word that no arms were hidden in the hotel; in all good faith a regiment marched by, and were instantly opened fire on from the windows by a machine-gun. The men burst in, and were met on the staircase by Commander Locker Lampson and several British officers, who succeeded in saving the women and children from rough handling and, to a certain degree, in controlling the men.

There was a curious scene at the opera one night. During an entr'acte half a dozen soldiers walked on to the stage, and, addressing the audience, their spokesman explained that his regiment now in Petrograd had been to the Front and had suffered very severely. They were now resting, but if subscriptions were forthcoming they might find it possible to fight again. The hat was then passed round by fairies from the chorus! Thus were we reminded of the Revolution and murdered generals floating in the canals, workers asking for a six-hour day, strikes and much singing of the *Marseillaise* all bore witness.

The great palaces are all deserted or confiscated for public purposes; their owners have either fled or else are prisoners.

The trouble is that instead of one clear impression of the Revolution one comes away with half a dozen contradictory ones.

I think that the truest view of the empress is that she worked unconsciously in enemy interests, partly owing to her submission to influences at court now admittedly German, but largely owing to her intense fear of the people. She was determined to hand on the power to her son undiminished, and was incapable of associating increased freedom with the conception of a powerful throne.

Of the *tsar's* loyalty there seems not the smallest doubt, but it is really tragic to think of the tremendous opportunity that man missed.

Lately there is some improvement reported in the attitude of the troops at the Front. Capital punishment has been abolished some time, and any attempt on the part of the officers to prevent fraternization with the enemy has hitherto usually ended fatally for the former. But a different case was reported the other day from the Riga Front. Some men caught fraternizing were court-martialled by their own Soldiers' Committee, marched out to no-man's-land, and there flogged in full view of the German troops. The punishment was severe. One man died, and four are now in hospital.

Hospital "stuff" is frightfully short all over Russia. England sends out a fair quantity, but the congestion at Archangel makes delivery very slow. At one of the poorer Petrograd hospitals bandages are changed once a fortnight! Discipline in hospital makes the well-brought-up British hair rise. The men come and go, stay or vanish at their own sweet wills, but as a rule it is the men who have been wounded who are ready to go on. In judging them one must remember that before the Revolution soldier's pay was 75 *kopeks* a month (less than 1s. in English money), and that they fought with no hope of leave, with little or no news from home, and, so I have been told, with the knowledge that in the event of disablement they would have to face the world again with a clean shirt, 10*rs.* (roughly 15s.) and perhaps a begging licence for all capital.

The other day Lady Georgina Buchanan was leaving one of the hospitals, where she had been visiting a convoy of maimed prisoners of war just returned from Germany. At the door a sister called her back, saying that one of the men, not having before realised that she was English, would like to speak to her. She found a man lying in bed. "Excellency," he said, "I want to thank you in all our names for the wonderful kindness shown to us by our British fellow-prisoners. Everything they had they shared with us."

CHAPTER 10

June

June 1st. In the Train. Haparanda-Stockholm.

We arrived at Torneo, the frontier town of Finland, about 12, and after luggage and Passport formalities were shipped across the river to Haparanda. Our luggage is everywhere let through without question, but the civilians have a bad time of it. At Haparanda a doctor hopefully inquired whether we were suffering from either smallpox or cholera.

We put our kit-bags on a truck and started to walk up to the station. A Swedish soldier insisted on carrying our bundles, talked to us in excellent English, and proved to have been educated at Oxford. Half-way to the station we passed a little church and cemetery. Here Russian prisoners returning home from Germany are buried when their strength fails them at the frontier. It is pretty tragic.

And now sadly—farewell to Holy Russia.

June 2nd. In the Train. Haparanda-Stockholm.

All day in the train. Attractive but quite "expected" country, and two nice women, one Russian and one English, in the carriage. Next door an extraordinarily amusing American. He sits in our midst most of the day, patting poor little Europe on the back, telling us tall stories, his plans past, present, and future, of his friends and his achievements, failing quite comically to understand the first thing about Russia, but always amusing and always good-tempered, with an unrivalled gift of expression. The most vital being I have met for months, and it has been fun coming across his as the first personality after ten months in Russia the Oriental.

The cleanliness of everything is quite marvellous; I already miss the "do as you please" attitude of back yonder. Here so many things are "*verboten.*"You may not sit on the coach steps or climb on the roof if you feel so inclined, you mayn't even be left behind if you want to. And spitting is considered a nasty habit. What would they say to the Russian soldier who, when the regimental doctor urged upon him the uses of a pocket handkerchief, replied: "Why should I keep a 'cabinet' in my pocket?"

The food is good, and bread tickets were issued to us on the frontier.

June 3rd. In the Train. Stockholm-Christiania.

Arrived at Stockholm early. A pouring wet Sunday, and nothing to do, so we filled up the time touring round the town on a tram, and eating and washing at the best hotel.

We are forced to associate with Germans—hungry brutes, glad enough to be rid of the Fatherland. In the smoking-room of the hotel there were men reading the Scandinavian papers, the *Berliner Tageblatt*, the *New York Herald*, the *Novoe Vremya* and *The Times*—and yet there was no murder!

We left about 9 p.m. The Russian(?) sister who tried to pump me as to when the boat left Bergen has disappeared.

June 4th. Christiania.

Arrived at Christiania about 11 a.m., and S. met us on the platform. We left our stuff at an hotel, and spent the rest of the day with her at the legation. Very hot. It is a most pleasant spot. We leave for Bergen early tomorrow.

June 5th. Bergen.

In the train all day and a wonderful journey. From hot Christiania through snow and ice back to the *fjords* and a lovely sunset—I just loved it. The only adventure was a broken bridge. We were made suddenly to disembark, and carry all our baggage over a roaring torrent, and then camp in a tremendous downpour of rain until such time as a train came to pick us up. We got to Bergen at 11 p.m., and were taken to lodge at a hospital for the night.

June 6th.

Free-born Bergen is on strike, hence a complete absence of carriages and trams. C., I, and two of the sisters from the hospital tottered the two miles to the consulate with all our luggage, and arrived in a most unbecoming state of heat. But we were quite comforted to hear that the boat was to leave this afternoon.

C. looted a sort of Lord Mayor's coach in her best Russian manner—the driver was so astonished that he became as wax—we hauled our kit-bags out of the customs and proceeded to the quay, leaving our fellow-travelling civilians to gnash their teeth and—wait. We found our boat, and a cabin and English sailors and a quite gorgeously nasty English tea.

The boat left amidst sympathetic and eternal farewells. And now, in the words of the gunner: "Ye can just go to yer-r bunks and sleep, for ye're safe as churches and ye'll be in A-berr-deen tomorrow after-r-noon." In other words—"*Je m'en fiche bien des Bosches.*"

June 7th. In the Train. Aberdeen-King's Cross.

Nothing will make me believe that Aberdeen is not the eighth wonder of the world and the most beautiful city on earth.

A History of the Scottish Women's
Hospitals
(Extract concerning service in the Balkans)

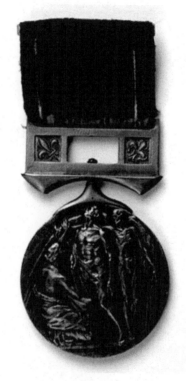

SCOTTISH WOMEN'S HOSPITALS
MEDAL

Contents

Introduction

No claim is made in the following history to a unique position for the Scottish Women's Hospitals. By many another organisation, started during the last five years, (as at time of first publication), the story of as great and as good work could be told. The material which formed the personnel of the S.W.H. was the everyday woman of the Empire, drawn from all classes.

Dr. Inglis, writing on the voyage to Russia, and describing an obstacle race on board ship, says:

I do like the modern British girl, with her love of outdoor sports, her energy, her resource, and her independence.

To this splendid product of the times, the modern British girl, with her high courage, her disregard of difficulties, and her beauty born of strength and health, who formed the rank and file of the units, was much of the success of the S.W.H. due. She was sent out by women of mature wisdom and experience, and she was led by some of the finest women in the Empire.

The story told in the following pages is given, almost entirely, in the words of the women who did the work. It was felt that this was the most certain way of obtaining a living narrative. It falls naturally into seven parts. An appreciation of Dr. Elsie Inglis stands in the middle, with chapters on each side describing the work with which she was most intimately connected.

It was the good fortune of the Scottish Women to be able to give to the French four years of uninterrupted service in France, and over three years in Salonika. With the exception of the first four months, the Scottish Women worked for the Serbian nation during the whole war, through all their changing fortunes With then they grappled with the dread typhus and overcame it; they accompanied them in the

Great Retreat; they tended their wounded and prisoners in Krushev-atz. and their refugees in Corsica; they followed them fighting through the Moglena Mountains; they strained to keep up with their victori-ous armies over crest after crest, in the "breathless rush" to Prilep, past Krushevatz and Kruguievatz (names dear to the Scottish Women), and at the rear of their armies they entered Belgrade, privileged to stand by them in their humiliation and to join in their triumph.

The work which fell to be performed by the Scottish Women's' Hospitals was varied. It ranged from the organisation of a baby show held in Corsica, amongst the Serbian Refugees, to helping to conduct an army division through the length of Russia.

By the courtesy of the Foreign Office in granting permission for its publication, the story of the diplomatic work done in Russia by the S.W.H. is told in this history for the first time. In the letter to Miss Mair giving this permission, Lord Curzon expressed his anxiety "to be of any assistance in the preparation of a history of the Scottish Wom-en's Hospitals, of whose heroic work he has the greatest admiration."

In a letter addressed to Mr. A. F. Whyte by the Secretary of State for War. Mr. Winston Churchill speaks of his admiration of the services performed by the Scottish Women's Hospitals in many fields through-out the war. He writes:

> The record of their work in Russia and Roumania lit up by the fame of Dr. Elsie Inglis, will shine in history. Their achieve-ments in France, in Serbia, in Greece, and in other theatres were no less valuable, and no body of women has won a higher repu-tation for organising power and for efficacy in works of mercy. It is a pleasure to me to remember that in the early days of the war I had the opportunity of furthering their efforts.

Sincere thanks are due not only to the Foreign Office, but also to all those who were asked, either for information with regard to the units or to contribute to the history, and who in every case responded with keenness and enthusiasm.

Miss S. E. S. Mair has given the chapter on "Our Chief": Miss Ed-ith Palliser undertook the whole of Part 4; while without the expert help of Miss Muriel Craigie, the *History* could not have taken shape.

The world is richer today because of the many heroic figures which have emerged from the wreckage left by the war: souls nobly efficient because they we're above the petty meannesses of life, humble and fearless, powerful with the power of self-sacrifice.

To this heroic band it will be the lasting pride of the Scottish Women that it was their privilege to contribute more than one; and also that the glorious service was theirs, of helping in their time of stress, men drawn without distinction from every one of the Allied Forces.

HOSPITALS

DESTINATION.	DATE.	C.M.O.
CALAIS	Dec. 1914–March 1915	Dr. ALICE HUTCHISON
ROYAUMONT	Dec. 1914–Feb. 1919	Miss IVENS
SERBIA	Dec. 1914–Jan. 1916	
1. KRAGUIEVATZ	Dec. 1914–Nov. 1915	{ Dr. INGLIS Dr. SOLTAU
2. VALJEVO	May 1915–Nov. 1915	Dr. HUTCHISON
3. MLADANOVATZ	May 1915–Nov. 1915	Dr. McGREGOR
4. LAZAROVATZ	Aug. 1915–Nov. 1915	Dr. HOLLWAY
TROYES	May 1915–Oct. 1915	{ Dr. McILROY Dr. SANDEMAN
SALONIKA	Dec. 1915–March 1919	Dr. McILROY
CORSICA	Dec. 1915–April 1919	{ Dr. BLAIR Dr. PHILLIPS Dr. COURTAULD Dr. MACPHAIL Dr. GUEST Dr. KEER
OSTROVO * With Transport Column attached	Aug. 1916–Nov. 1918	{ Dr. BENNETT Dr. DE GARIS
VRANJA	Nov. 1918	Dr. EMSLIE
RUSSIA With Transport Column attached	Aug. 1916–Nov. 1917	Dr. INGLIS
SERBIA With Transport Column attached	Feb. 1918–Feb. 1919	Dr. BENSON
SALLANCHES	Feb. 1918–March 1919	{ Dr. MACPHAIL Dr. BULLOCK

* Later this Column, under Miss Dillon, was attached to the 1st Serbian Army.

PART 1

CHAPTER 1

The Scottish Federation

Europe was submerged in darkness. War, horrible and hateful, occupied the minds and hearts of the people.

Righteous though the cause of the Allies was, the warfare entailed was beyond words terrible. The darkness grew denser, but in the surrounding gloom, throughout the wide zone of war, shone the beacon lights of the buildings thing the Red Cross flag.

The spirits of hate and love, cruelty and mercy, walked side by side on the battlefields. Civilised nations at war-what a strange picture they present! The peoples march to the battlefields organised to the utmost limit for the work of slaughter, organised, too, to the same extent for the work of healing and saving those that have escaped alive from the carnage. With all the finished skill they can command, equipped with the finest science of their day, they use against each other the most terrible engines of war, till men lie wounded, and maimed, and blinded, and deafened, and then they gather together those wounded, and maimed, and blind, and deaf, and, again armed with the finest science of the day, expend the most tender care in the endeavour to resuscitate the dying, and to heal the wounded.

The organisation for healing is no less finished and complete than that for destruction.

It is about five o'clock in the afternoon, when the light fails, that the worst hour in the hospital begins. The dim lamps are lighted, and people begin to fall over things. Also, this is the hour, it seems to me, when men feel pain most, when the wounded in beds and on the floor begin to cry out. How they suffer! Here is a young boy with his eyes shot out, and several beds in a row contain men with head wounds, the result of bursting shrapnel overhead. And there are other cases too pitiful to describe; and men who have lost their reason: and men moaning for morphia; and a baby of three years with both his legs broken, and a little bandaged hand at which he looks in wonder.

It isn't a good time—war is not a merry picnic. Blood-covered mattresses and pillows are carried out into the courtyard. There is always a great pile of rags and bandages being burnt outside. A curious smell pervades everything.

In the midst of it all, doctors and nurses keep their heads, and are never flurried, never less than careful and attentive. They sit up all night, and in the noisy daytime get but little sleep; they have become inured to seeing death and suffering without being hardened by it, and their patience is admirable.[1]

A visitor to an operating theatre in the war zone might readily imagine he was back again in one of the famous hospitals of London or Edinburgh, Paris or Petrograd. There he would meet expert surgeons and physicians, highly trained nurses, and alert and skilful orderlies, and he would find an equipment of instruments and appliances of the latest design and the finest material. If he could extend his visit through France and Belgium, Italy and Austria, Germany, Russia and Serbia, wherever battles were waged, behind the long line of fighting he would find the long line of those well-equipped hospitals, where the highest medical and surgical skill in Europe was at the disposal of the poor sufferers.

But amongst them all, at points in Europe far distant from each other, he would come upon a certain number of hospitals with a feature distinguishing them from all the others. They are evidently equally well equipped, the staff of doctors and assistants is as expert and capable and the strain of the work is met by the same smooth and rapid efficiency.

What, then, is the distinguishing mark? It is this—they are "manned" from end to end by women, and women only. Women drivers take the ambulance car, into the firing line, women stretcher-bearers lift the wounded, and place them in the ambulances, women doctors await them in the hospital. It is women who perform the operations, remaining at work in the theatres, it may be sometimes thirty-six and fifty hours at a stretch. Women nurses and orderlies attend the patients in the wards, women cook the entire food required by the hospital,

---

1. *A Woman's Diary of the War* by S. Macnaughten.

and women bury amputated limbs and carry on disinfecting and other sanitary work. And he would find this too—that the scheme for these hospitals had originated in the brain of a woman, and that they were equipped and controlled by a women's society in Britain.

★★★★★★

In a small room up a long flight of stairs in 2 St. Andrew Square, Edinburgh, a woman, already well known in the medical world, realised in a flash what an all important part women could take in the war. As Dr. Elsie Inglis sat in the offices of the Scottish Federation of Women's Suffrage Societies, she saw in imagination the army of women, skilled and unskilled, who only needed organising to be brought into line with the most efficient service the nation knew. To carry out this organising she set to work on the very outbreak of war. She had at her back the women of the Federated Suffrage Societies of Scotland, and farther afield the whole force of the National Union of Women's Suffrage Societies throughout the United Kingdom.

How the scheme of the hospitals was born and grew can be gleaned from the minutes of the Federation.

The growth of the idea during one Committee meeting is recorded for us in the minutes of the meeting held on 12th August—the first Federation Committee after war broke out.

> Dr. Inglis proposed that the Federation should give organised help to Red Cross work
>
> Miss Mair proposed that St. George's School, Melville Street, should be applied for and equipped as a hospital.
>
> Dr Inglis proposed that Melville Street School be equipped as a hospital *staffed entirely by women*—if not required at home to be sent abroad.

And so the scheme was launched. "*Silver and gold had we none,*" the Scottish federation might have said, "but such as we have we give to our nation now." Enthusiasm, courage, undaunted faith, these were the gifts they offered. The coffers of the Federation were not over full. What Suffrage Society ever had them overflowing? The Suffrage Societies were a body of women well organised, growing in numbers, imbued with "the long range point of view," and full of determination and belief in their cause, but certainly not a body receiving much backing from the public, financially or in any other way. However, once more, the history of the Scottish Women's Hospitals was to prove the fact that money is not everything. Courage, undaunted faith, and clear vision are of more value. Of these, there are no lack in the members who formed the Committee of the Scottish Federation, though even there "some doubted." When it was stated that a thousand pounds would need to be raised to equip the one unit thought of in these early days, a member, it is reported, dropped her head and moaned, "We might as well ask for a million at once!"

It was found impossible to obtain the houses in Melville Street for a hospital, and accordingly it was decided to offer the unit to the War Office. This offer was declined. It was then resolved to offer the unit to one of the Allies. On 20th August just eight days after their first meeting, the following letter was sent to the Embassies of Belgium, France and Russia.

The Scottish Federation
Women's Suffrage Societies Edinburgh
20th August 1914

To His Excellency the Ambassador for ——

Sir,—A number of Scottish women have it in their minds to fit out a Red Cross Hospital for use at the seat of war, and to offer it to one of the governments involved in the war. It is possible that you could supply us with some information as to the position with regard to the Red Cross Service in connection with the —— troops on the Continent? The scheme is only in its initial stages at present, but we should be very glad to know whether your government is already more than sufficiently equipped in connection with its hospital service—

Yours Faithfully   Elsie Maud Inglis,
Hon. Secretary

The minutes of the Federation meeting held on 3rd October, supply the next point of interest though all the intervening ones mark the steady progress of the scheme. On the one hand it is evident that plans have now matured, and the details of the units have taken fixed shape; while on the other we find that the scheme, hitherto supported only by the branches of the Federation in Scotland, is now to receive recognition across the border.

Dr. Inglis reported in her estimate that a thousand pounds would be sufficient to pay salaries of one unit of 100 beds for six months.[2] Each unit to consist of four doctors (two seniors

---

2. It was owing to the number of voluntary workers that Dr Inglis' estimate was put at so low a figure as £1000.

and two juniors), ten trained nurses, six dressers, two cooks, an administrator, and a clerk. Suggested that one unit might go to Serbia, where need is very great."

A letter was read from Mrs. Fawcett agreeing that an appeal for funds for the Hospital Scheme should be made at the .National Union meeting on 20th October in the Kingsway Hall, London.

The funds were still low. On 13th October Dr Inglis, writing to Mrs. Fawcett, says:

In answer to your questions, first as to the amount of money collected, up to date we have collected £115 with all the help *Common Cause* has given to us, Tomorrow our appeal goes broadcast over Scotland, ten thousand copies, and I hope to be able to report progress in a day or two. . .We are getting a lot of offers of voluntary service.

October 20th stands out as a great date in the history of the S.W.H. On that day Dr. Inglis spoke at the Kingsway Hall, in London, on behalf of the hospitals. Since that date thousands of meetings in aid of the S.W.H. have been held all over the British Empire. Miss Burke in America has addressed audiences of any number up to ten thousand. Her speeches have aroused unparalleled enthusiasm, as the resulting contributions show. Mrs. Abbott in India and Australia has addressed meetings which have been prolific in interest and in funds, one meeting alone in Calcutta resulting in thirteen thousand pounds. Meetings have been held in every sort of hall and drawing-room in every part of the United Kingdom, but friends of the S.W.H. will always recall with peculiar interest that meeting held on the 20th of October in the capital of the Empire, at which for the first time the scheme for taking aid to the fighting men of the Allies by hospitals staffed entirely by women was made known by the founder of the S.W.H.

From that date money began to flow in, in a steady stream, until at the end of the war the sum of £449,000 had been reached. On 20th October a letter from the Headquarters of the National Union says:

As the result of your stirring appeal at the meeting at Kingsway Hall we are receiving at this office a large number of inquiries about the Scottish Hospital.

Mrs. Fawcett, who had written to the *Times* regarding the project, writes on 7th November 1914 to Dr. Inglis:

I think your fund must be well over three thousand. But we must go on—the more we get the better, for I feel quite certain that one thousand per unit is not enough. The Finance Department of the National Union wrote last night that letters and cheques were still arriving by every post. I am so glad.

On her return to Scotland, Dr. Inglis formed on 31st October, out of the Federation and some of her personal friends, the Scottish Women's Hospitals Committee, with Mrs. James T. Hunter of Glasgow as Chairman. It was decided at this meeting, that the uniform was to be the "hodden grey," with Gordon tartan facings. Dr. Inglis next sent out the organisers of the Federation on their first missionary journey for the S.W.H. They were sent broadcast, as the appeal had been, all over Scotland, and told to appeal for twenty thousand pounds. They went, carrying the gospel of the dawning era of the recognition of women's work in the welfare of the nation. One dwells with pride on the memory of these first missionaries of the S.W.H. To them it was a "great adventure." The scheme for which they had to appeal was daring and fascinating in its originality, and with them rested the responsibility of "setting the heather alight." That supporters of the hospitals were soon found all over the world is a witness to the way they did their work.

For the S.W.H., accepted in the first instance by the N.U.W.S.S.[3] and remembering proudly all through the years of their existence this parentage, "have formed a wonderful rallying-point for women of every shade of political opinion—non-suffragist and anti-suffragist alike pouring their money into the common funds and giving their personal service." Several of the largest subscriptions in the early days were from prominent anti-suffragists. A personal friend of Dr. Inglis', who had strongly disapproved of her Suffrage work, in sending her a cheque, wrote:

I am glad you are doing something useful at last!

On 21st November, five thousand four hundred and four pounds had been subscribed, and in that month the colleges of Girton and Newnham had offered to raise fifteen hundred pounds to equip another unit. On 9th December the funds in hand were over six thousand five hundred and seven pounds.

---

3. National Union of Women's Suffrage Societies.

CHAPTER 2

The Units Forming

During the months of September, October, and November, whilst the funds were increasing from one hundred and fifteen to over six thousand pounds, the actual preparation of the units was proceeding apace—the idea of a single unit had long been abandoned, and the number of hospitals was to be limited only by the amount of money subscribed. The first emissary of the S.W.H., in the person of Dr. Alice Hutchison, went over to France on 7th November 1914. A postcard from her of that date to Dr. Inglis is worth preserving:

> Dear Dr. Inglis,—Dr. Clark wrote to you as I was leaving home yesterday. My day was an appalling rush. I cross to Calais to-day. I am not sure with whom to hunt the coast tomorrow— Dunkirk, Gravelines, etc.—for a suitable building. There is not a barn left at Calais for wounded pouring in. I must dash up to Edinburgh if possible on my return, as I came to Harburg with a fortnight's luggage. If it's impossible, I'll manage somehow—I am delighted to do this trip for you.

On that same date the following letter was received from the French Embassy:

> *Ambassade de France,*
> *A Londres*, 7th November 1914
> The Secretary to the French Embassy presents his compliments to the President of the Scottish Women's Hospital, and begs to thank her for her kind offer of the 5th inst. With regard to a new arrangement between the French War Office and the British Red Cross, all offers for hospitals abroad are to be examined by the British Red Cross, 83 Pall Mall.

On 8th November Dr. Seton Watson wired:

Hutchison, going over to France for an indefinite period, 'hunting the coast' so gaily for a building for the S.W.H., with only a fortnight's luggage with her, is a daughter of a medical missionary in the north of India, whose fame as a devoted doctor and a fearless traveller has spread far and wide amongst the people of the Western Himalayas. Anyone who knew him could have no difficulty in tracing the source of the intrepid courage, the unfailing resourcefulness, and the devotion to work found in the daughter.

Dr. Hutchison will be often met in these pages. Dr. Inglis' tribute to her was:

Anyone working under Alice Hutchison once is always ready to do so again.

At the end of November Dr. Inglis gave in her first report to the S.W.H. committee as to what had been done since the inaugural meeting on 12th August.

The work is already beginning to open out its various ways, and the proposed hospital come to shew the committee shewn provide the medical personnel, beds linen & dressings for a hospital ship which is to ply between ...... & Dover

Before the Committee undertake any further scheme however they would wish to be to see the beds which are now ready at work, & the Canteens contemplated to supply refreshment men to Deepage. They would also like to see how much more money comes in for their ventures.

Offers of service still come in daily a gift of ...... out of hospital requirements
The Committee desire to thank their ......

...... have been laid down. ...... that production ...... by the late rooms erected at the disposal of the committee by the Insurance Business Company have already .... being ...... at ...... the Bible .... these are of

CHAPTER 3

Calais

On 19th November 1914, just three months after the Scottish Women had offered a hospital for service abroad. Dr. Hutchison and Sister Linton went over to Calais in answer to Dr. Depage's request, to see in what way the Scottish Women could help the Belgians. For a few days there was quiet, and not much prospect of any hard work. Then typhoid broke out in the Belgian Army and Calais was taxed to its utmost to meet the emergency. On 5th December Dr. Hutchison was put in charge of a typhoid annexe to Dr. Depage's hospital and with Dr. Phillips and ten fully trained nurses had three months of unceasing work until the epidemic came to an end.

The following quotations taken from Dr Hutchison's letters to her many friends during these three month's work in the typhoid annexe:

19th November
Dr. Depage's hospital is being organised by the Queen of the Belgians, who sent Dr. Depage to try and bring order out of the existing chaos. He is their big surgeon, hence her choice. I understand it is an entity by itself, neither under the Red Cross nor War Office.

15th December, 1912
I feel that a letter of some sort must be sent off today, or you will all soon have forgotten my existence. Well, on Saturday, 5th December. I was sent for to Dr. Depage's private room, where I found two generals resplendent in gold lace and other adornments befitting their high station, to whom Dr. Depage presented me as—'this is the doctor of whom I spoke to you,' and there and then it was fixed up that Dr. Depage should give up

his annexe of eighty beds for typhoid work, and that I should work there with my ten nurses and Dr. Phillips. I quite realised that the generals were not dying to have us, but I determined that they should arrive at the stage of being loath to lose us, by before long. I stipulated for two days' grace to get my nurses over.[1]

The two days' grace was accorded in word but not in deed, for on Sunday morning, when I was busy doing some dressing at Jeanne d'Arc (Dr. Depage's hospital), an orderly came to say that five cases had been admitted to the Rue Archimède (the annexe). From then on they simply poured in, and Sister Linton and I had no further need to complain of an idle existence. On my next letter I shall tell you how we run the place and how I did many things in those early days which I never dreamed of doing.

22nd December.

Dear Everybody,—I have sat down to give you a description of this place and of our work here, as it would doubtless interest you to know the conditions under which we are working.

The building where we work was a school, and the house we live in was the schoolmistress's house. We are nearly on the edge of the town, surrounded on both hands by patches of waste-ground, and with a large factory at the back of us. Arrived at our big wooden doorway, you ring the bell and step into a covered courtyard—the door to the right leads into our house, and that on the left leads into the five schoolrooms, now our wards. The wards all open into one another in a straight line, and we have ten beds in each.

Our dwelling-house could hardly be more bare than it is; but it is a barren simplicity, not tawdriness. In the early days we had no servant, and Sister Linton turned to like a perfect brick and ran the house and kitchen. Now we have a very nice woman, a Frenchwoman called Jeanne, whose husband was killed at the Front in October, and who has in consequence to support herself and her baby. I think somehow Jeanne will soon become an indispensable part of our *ménage*, and one of our pleasantest memories after we have gone.

---

1. The remaining nurses left Edinburgh next day, 6th December, arriving at Calais within forty hours of their start.

The first two days here, when Sister Linton and I were alone, remain in my mind as a nightmare. All day long the ambulance drove up, and patients were carried in on stretchers, and ward after ward filled up with appalling rapidity Sister Linton and I, with the help of one or two young Belgian priests, ran about doing what we could in the way of sponging, feeding, etc., with, if my memory does not play me false, an occasional dash in three different directions at the same time, to prevent delirious patients from getting out of bed.

We have several young Belgian priests as orderlies, and find them excellent. Their training seems to have developed in them a spirit of discipline, submissiveness, and devotion to duty which results in first-class work. Of them all, however, Brother Michael is the favourite. We have also a young parish priest. Monsieur l'Aumonier, who makes a round of the wards every day, distributing literature and words of consolation to those who are not delirious, and granting a few words of absolution to any whose condition is reported to him as critical. Monsieur l'Aomonier is quite a nice young man, but he isn't a patch on Monsieur l'Abbeé, the portly priest of Ambulance Jeanne d'Arc.

I am being splendidly supported in the work here by Dr. Phillips and my ten Scottish nurses. The latter are working like bricks, and I am glad to think they will have some relaxation on Christmas night, when we have been invited to dine and dance at the Sophie Berthelet, the English hospital here."

Extract from a letter to Dr. Inglis, written after Dr. Inglis' visit of inspection:

It is good of you to be so appreciative of the work here. It would be nice to feel when we leave that we had sensibly advanced the whole position of women by our little contribution of work here.

4th January.

Whenever one gets irritated or vexed with the Belgians one feels oneself pulled up by the realisation of the painfully unique position they are in, having no claim to any but the smallest corner of their country, and many of them having no knowledge of the whereabouts of even their wives and children. When Christmas Day came I wished them the only wish which I felt was not a mere humbug—I wished them the following Christmas in their own country, a country completely freed from German rule. How different it is walking through our wards now from what it was even two weeks ago! Then the wards were so silent that it was like a house of the dead. The only interludes to the heavy silence were the noisy declamations of delirious patients.

Now it seems as if a magician's wand had touched the place, and all is noise and chatter and brightness.

The epidemic is a severe one, with many grave complications. One never has a dull moment.

30th January 1915.

Dear Everybody.—It is some time since I sent united news to you, so I must try to finish this letter tonight, and get it posted tomorrow. Most weeks here the days are so much alike and one hardly notices their flight. The washerwoman appears one morning with the household napery, and one realises it is Sunday, or she appears the following morning with the personal washing, and one realises it is Monday. So the days pass into weeks and the weeks into months, and one begins to wonder whether the months will stretch into years, and still find this small band of British women at its post in Calais.

I am glad to be able to report one big advance in our arrangements. A camp for convalescent typhoids is in full swing now at Ruchard, about 26 miles from Tours. So we shall always be able to empty and fill very regularly, and so make the most of our fifty beds. There is one drawback to Ruchard, that it means twenty-seven hours' train journey, so that we cannot send patients away till they are thoroughly fit.

The first clear-out took place soon after my last letter was sent, and first clear-outs, especially in wartime, are rather outstanding events, even more so than the arrival of the washerwoman! The sister of one of my wards got a most delicately and quaintly expressed note (in English) written by an English-speaking patient in an attempt to give utterance to the surcharged feelings of two Flamands. As the motor set off for the station, after the usual snorting and puffing, my thoughts were back in Bulgaria.[2] I saw once again the long line of bullock carts, packed with

---

2. Previous to 1914, Dr. Hutchison had worked in Bulgaria in the first Balkan War.

convalescent wounded, setting slowly in motion with many a creak and groan, allowing ample time for renewed handshakes and parting injunctions. Memories sometimes come like benedictions.

We have been very busy, and I have been so grateful for the splendid way in which our nurses have tackled the work. Some of them are having considerable success in training the '*Frères*' to be of some real use in the wards, even in some cases to wash up a patient and change his sheets. You can understand that with several delirious or unconscious patients on hand there is bound to be a tremendous lot of that sort of work to do.

I must tell you about Céline, who for a few days added a warm touch of colour to the ward life. I introduce you to her as abruptly as she appeared on the scene. On going into the ward one evening, I found one of my favourite patients, who had been, as the French say, 'within two fingers of death,' impatiently awaiting me with a telegram in his hands. I read the following pathetic lines: 'I am at Dieppe. Can I see thee if I come? Kisses Céline.'

Then had I to wage a fierce warfare, using all my artillery, big and small, against the terrible bugbear, '*La Loi Militaire.' La Loi Militaire* says that no typhoid fever patient may receive visitors, and refuses to make an exception in the case of a poor little woman who takes fright on hearing that her husband is at Calais, because 'she knew everyone who went to Calais had enteric,' who then takes her courage in her hands and risks everything to get past that barbed-wire barrier which now marks the Belgian-Dutch frontier. To leave openly in the train is impossible, as no Belgian is allowed to leave the country, so a weary tramp across bogs and fields has to be undertaken, till an isolated spot is found, where patrol sentries are scarce, and where one finally escapes by throwing oneself flat and crawling under the barbed-wire.

Many arrive in Holland with their clothes hopelessly torn, but as Céline proudly said, 'I had the sense to put on my old ones.' Well in the end, I managed to silence the enemy's guns; but when Céline swept in on us as fresh and vigorous as a moorland wind, I realised that I had wasted power, for Céline with her charming smile would have swept past any general in creation. When her husband realised what she had faced to get here, he said, '*Quelle folie*;' while I added, '*Quelle folie glorieuse!*'

The day Céline left I received a charming little basket, daintily arranged with a mixture of Parma violets and ordinary violets—a huge yellow bow on one side and a small rosette of the Belgian colours below it. Accompanying it was a delicately worded little note expressing some of Céline's innermost feelings. Dear Céline, she will always be with me as a charming and gracious memory: and I never so regretted our disuse of 'thou' as when I heard her suddenly break off in the middle of a vivacious account of her adventures, then touch her husband's hand and say, ;To think that thou wast nearly dead, and now I have thee safely here.'

You can see that we have much to cheer us, but we have also much to sadden us. A lovely big schoolboy of a creature was brought in one day who had left school in July, and was fighting in the trenches in august. There was not a life we longed more to save, so as to be able to send him back in the vigour of his youth and his boyish beauty to the '*mère et Hélène*' whom he spoke of so incessantly, but . . . . we failed. It was at least comfort to be able to send them word that their Henri had not lacked for a mother touch from the women who had looked after him.

One night a man was brought in, already noisily delirious and drumming out his own funeral march in loud and resonant tones. Again and yet again he rolled it out with an intermixture of comic camp songs till the eeriness got too much for us. Forty-eight hours later he slipped out as silently as he had come in boisterously.

I think there is no harm in me telling you that I have been greatly comforted this week to find that our hospital has the lowest percentage mortality for enteric in Calais.

We all keep wonderfully well, and I hope we shall continue to do so. It is difficult to believe one is in Calais, the all-pervading dampness of it is so reminiscent of dear old Scotland! French people, however, assure me that they cannot within their memory recall such another damp winter.

In March 1915 the epidemic had been overcome, and Dr. Hutchison and her nurses returned to Britain. The annexe was one of the few hospitals in Calais where fully trained British Sisters were to be found upon the staff. Of the trained British nurse it has been said, that during the war she was "worth her weight not in gold, but in diamonds."

According to official returns, the death-rate in the annexe was lower than in any other hospital in Calais.

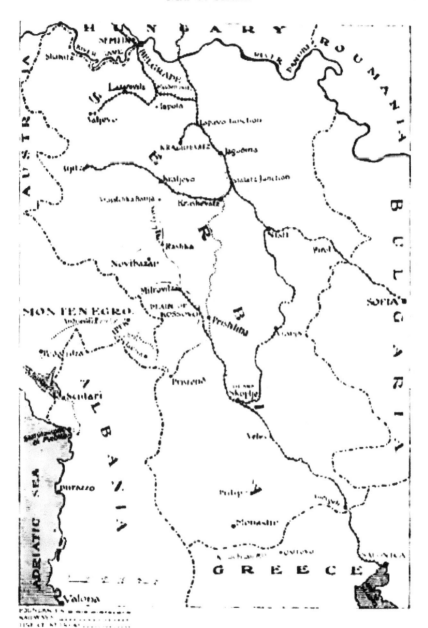

CHAPTER 1

Introductory

By the seventh century the people occupying the region of
modern Serbia were Slavonic in origin, and it was their destiny
to retain the customs and desires of the Slav people throughout
all the vicissitudes which came to them. From the arid Russian
Steppes they had reached a land of surpassing beauty. Four great
mountain ranges made junction within its boundaries, and at
least four-fifths of the total area is mountainous. Swiftly flowing torrents pass through beautifully wooded defiles, giving to
the artist a sense of the picturesque and to the soldier visions
of strategic positions making successful defence easy, and to
the practical man offering a manifestation of unlimited power
waiting for adaptation.

In some degree the Serbian has developed all three sides in his
character, though his commercial instincts have not been so
apparent as his military and artistic capacities. The temperate
climate produces luxuriant foliage and a wonderful vegetation.
The wildness of the Serbian Highlands has tended to evolve
a hardy race of mountaineers, whose warlike proclivities have
never been allowed to rest through any period of prolonged
peace.[1]

It took four centuries for these loosely organised tribes of the lower Danube to be formed into a nation under their king, Stephen Voislav. The centuries had been full of wars with neighbouring tribes and
nations. Stephen Voislav was a descendant of one of the most notable
men in Serbian history, John Vladimir:

---

1. The quotations are from *The Story of Serbia*, by Leslie F. Church.

With a mysterious dignity, reminding one of the ancient priest-king Melchisedek, he flits across the broken century and fills its hollow years with a fragrant presence, kingly and not altogether unworthy of a saint. For the leader of a warlike race to have earned the character of a peaceful prince, full of honour and saintliness. would be remarkable in any period of history. The fact that John Vladimir survived the deathly silence of those times sets one speculating as to the greatness of the man.

Serbian history is full of heroes such as this—men with a strange mixture of warrior and saint in their composition.

From the middle of the fourteenth century the oncoming of the Turkish power became the real menace to Serbia. In 1389 the Battle of Kossovo was fought, in which the Serbians were completely crushed. After this defeat there was one brief temporary time of relief or Serbia: an outstanding personality arose in the person of John Hunyadi, who was called "The White Knight of Wallachia." He led many brilliant campaigns against the Turks.

Brilliant as these campaigns were, they were not sufficient to sap the immense resources of the Ottoman Empire. By July 1456 the Turks had again invested Belgrade, and the most highly organised plans of siege were put into action. For the last time John Hunyadi came to the rescue. By the most amazing and courageous strategy he relieved the beleaguered city. His little force penetrated the far-flung Turkish lines, established itself in Belgrade. and finally sallied forth with amazing audacity, to the complete discomfiture of the besiegers. Seldom in military annals does one read of a more valiant and impertinent success. Through the wonder, and the terror, of the pall of smoke, that hung over the lines of the new Ottoman artillery, two figures stood out sublimely heroic. John Hunyadi, with bared sword and bright armour, charged side by side with John of Capistrano the Minorite in dull habit but with crucifix raised fearlessly above the din of battle. In utter confusion the Turkish hordes fled. Amidst the rejoicing over this last great victory John Hunyadi died in August 1456. As far as Serbia was concerned the end had come.

For more than four long centuries she lay under the rule of Turkey. But never through all that dark period were the Turks able "to penetrate the remaining Serbs with their customs, their religion, or

137

with fear."

Wherever Serbs were found—in Hungary, in Bosnia, in Dalmatia, or Montenegro—they were singing the *Pesnias* or national songs, which reminded them alternately of the glory of Dushan and the shame of Kossovo. If they dwelt fugitives in the heart of the mountains: if they remained on sufferance in an alien land, or if they slept in the camps of European armies, in whose ranks they were soldiers, they never forgot they were Serbians. The wonderful compelling national poetry with its haunting music was the common property and prized possession of every Serb, whatever his present lot might be. This bond coupled with their loyalty to the Serbian Church, kept them spiritually a nation though they were separated by miles or centuries from its practical reality

And so they continued to hold together, clinging tenaciously to their yearning for freedom. Early in 1800 Kara George (Black George) arose. He was chosen their leader by the Serbian refugees, and carried all before him.

He started the revolt against the Turkish rule, which ended after many years of struggle in 1866, when the last Turkish soldier was turned out of the forts of Serbia. "The Soul of Serbia, immortal as it was, had burst its bonds at last, and soared upwards singing."

A strange people truly, mystical and warlike, tenacious and lovable—difficult to be understood by the practical nations of Europe—but surely easy of comprehension by another small nation living in a mountainous land, also mystical and warlike, and tenacious!

On 28th July 1914 Austria declared war on Serbia. The next day Russia was forced into mobilising, and Europe prepared for its greatest conflict. It was planned that the beginnings of the Great War should be in Serbia.

The forces of the Dual Empire massed themselves upon the banks of the Danube—their object was the punishment of Serbia. For the small nation just emerging from two previous wars, what hope was there? Their hope lay in the spirit of their forefathers. This spirit it was that, animating the men of Serbia, led them to victory, and at the Battle of the Ridges defeated their enemy. The unexpected had happened, and "the punitive expedition" hurried back to the Danube. From the scandalously filthy and overcrowded hospitals the Austrians left behind them there sprang the awful scourge of typhus. But even before the epidemic, which began in January 1915, swept over the land, Serbia had well-nigh plumbed the depth of suffering.

Thousands of wounded men, Austrian and Serb alike, choked to the doors every available house, and these temporary hospitals were found all over the country. The conditions created by these masses of wounded became a problem too vast to be solved by the handful of Serbian doctors. "Send us where we are most needed" was always the insistent demand of the Dr. Inglis. In the destination of the second unit of the Scottish Women's Hospitals this condition was fulfilled, for right into the heart of this distressed little nation went the Scottish Women in January 1915, taking their place in the "long-drawn-out battle" against wounds and fever and death.

CHAPTER 2

January–April, 1915

The long-drawn out battle against fever, in which no woman played the coward, and no woman asked to come away.

—Dr. Elsie Inglis.

During the fortnight in December 1914 when the women at Royaumont were at their work of cleaning the abbey the 2nd Unit of the S.W.H. sailed from Southampton under Dr. Eleanor Soltan, bound for the stricken land of Serbia.

When[1] we sailed, the position of Serbia seemed hopeless. Belgrade, the capital, had fallen, and the last news we received before sailing was that the Serbian Army. Lacking food and ammunition, was falling steadily back before the Austrian invasion. While we were in the Mediterranean the morning wireless to our troopship contained the news of a great Serbian victory, and on our arrival at Salonika the news was confirmed, so when we reached Serbia the country was almost free from the enemy, and King Peter had held a service of thanksgiving in the Cathedral of Belgrade. So much has happened in the course of the last few years that this battle, one of the most brilliant exploits of the Great War, has been rather lost sight of. It is known in Serbia as the Battle of the Ridges, and was complete in every way.

At Salonika the hospital got orders to entrain for Kraguievatz, in the north of Serbia, where help was urgently needed, and

---

1. The following account of the arrival of the S.W. H. in Kraguievatz is by Mr. William Smith of Aberdeen, who went out with Dr. Soltan's Unit as Transport Officer. He did yeoman service for the Scottish Women in Serbia. To his pen we also owe the story, given later, of one of the parties in the Great Retreat.

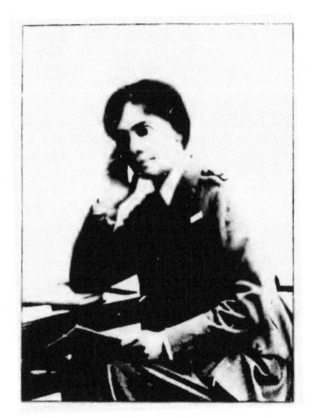

Dr. Eleanor Soltan

we left Salonika the morning after our arrival there. Our first stopping-place was Nish and it was well that we paused there, as it gave the doctors and staff some idea of the big job they would have to tackle at Kraguievatz. On arrival at the station we were met by the Army Authorities, and after breakfast we were taken to see the largest hospital in the town

As we approached the building we passed a great number of bullock wagons laden with wounded from the battle which was now nearing its close. The hospital was full to overflowing, and the wounded then arriving were being placed on the road and hospital yard (which was inches deep in mud), until other accommodation could be found for them. These ox wagons had taken several days and nights to the journey, and you can imagine the suffering of the wretched men with fractured limbs and worse injuries. Many died on the journey, and their bodies were left by the roadside. A few doctors and orderlies were doing what they could to relieve the suffering, but the doctors were few and the patients all too many, and they often waited their turn for hours in the cold winter day before they found shelter. But if the scene outside the hospital was a pitiful one, within the doors it was a thousand times worse, and I shall never forget the scene of misery, suffering and desolation we found there.

One of the largest buildings in the country was full to overflowing. Every inch of space was occupied—it was impossible to pass between the beds, for the poor patients were mostly lying on the floor, some on hay and straw, and others on the bare stone or wooden floors. Sick and wounded lay crowded together—men who had just undergone the amputation of limbs; men in the grip of typhoid, dysentery, or frostbite; men dying—some were dead. So close together were they lying that one patient could not move without disturbing his neighbour. Numbers had been lying there with their wounds undressed for a week or more, and the slightest wound, through lack of attention, often cost a man a limb, and sometimes his life.

Under such conditions many died of sheer neglect alone. The few doctors and nurse's were overwhelmed, and working night and day against fearful odds and with few or no appliances or medical stores. One surgeon told me that he had been several days without chloroform, and even major operations had been carried on without the aid of anaesthetics. Worst of all there was no means of ventilating these dreadful wards. The atmosphere was terrible—fit breeding-ground for the plague, which was about to descend on this already sorely stricken people. Some three weeks afterwards, in the midst of all this misery, confusion, and neglect, came typhus fever in the most virulent form, and before the authorities could do anything to check the plague, it had spread from one end of the country to the other. When the awful condition of Serbia became known, help was sent from almost every country in Europe and after three or four months' strenuous fighting the epidemic was gradually got under, but not before it had carried off between seventy and eighty thousand of the population.

The doctors and nurses of the S.W.H., inured to all manner of human suffering and more or less prepared for working under bad conditions, were, I think, struck dumb with the horror of it all, and there was no lack of food for thought during the rest of our journey from Nish to Kraguievatz.

We arrived at Kraguievatz the following morning and one of the many hospitals in the town was handed over to the Scottish Unit. It was much in the same condition as the one we saw at Nish the previous day, and which I have just described, but the whole staff set to, and in a week the place was transfigured. We had brought everything necessary in the way of equipment, oven to bedsteads, blankets, and clothing of all kinds, and we were not a little proud of our hospital when everything had been set going. Our patients were both Serbian and Austrian soldiers, friend and enemy lying side by side, seemingly on excellent terms with each other.

One by one the wards were emptied, cleaned, and whitewashed, the equipment was unpacked, and the patients, washed and tidied, were tucked up comfortably in the clean beds, with their bright red coverlets. The men's gratitude knew no bounds. The unit had gone out with an equipment for 100 beds; they had to take over 250 patients immediately on arrival.

Kraguievatz, January 1915,
Patients[1] were sent to us in batches until our wards were full,

---

1. The following extracts are from letters by different members of the staff to the committee.

and we still get them at intervals when we discharge convales-cents. They come from other hospitals in town, not fresh from the Front, as there has been no fighting for some time lately. They come to us in a terrible condition, having had absolutely no nursing. You can imagine from this, perhaps, what the hospitals are like. It is really not the Serbians' fault. The whole country is one immense hospital—doctors, Serbs and prisoners alike work all day merely to get the dressings done, and the drugs given out. There is no attempt at nursing—no Serbian women are trained for it, and they have become apathetic during their three wars. Many are refugees struggling to keep some sort of a house together.

You must realise, too, that the patients are no slum dwellers, but hate dirt and this utter discomfort. They are splendid men, magnificent even when they are dying of fever, but it is a most dreadful waste of fine human beings. . . . Hundreds and hundreds of nurses and doctor, are needed for Serbia, but especially nurses. . . . .

You see we are in a very sad country, but it is the pluckiest country in Europe, without exception. Here they are with their best men perishing on every side and they make no complaint, and never think for a moment of giving in, though the Austrians may be down on them yet. Austria has treated them abominably, and yet they are not bitter. Their prisoners get the same treatment—miserable though it is—as their own men do. Serbia is as proud as it is possible to be, and does not want other countries to pity her. She is a grand little country, and we all love her already, but she is desolate with her three wars. Why, we have men in our hospital almost boys, who proudly show their three scars—Turkish, Bulgar, and now Austrian.

Well, we are settled here in the crown prince's house, and, al-though crowded, are very much more comfortable than we expected to be. The hospital is five minutes walk away, and we have about 250 patients. . . . Their wounds are awful, and many of them just come in to die. They have been so crowded, too, in the last hospitals, that there is much fever We however, have kept free of it, you will be glad to learn. The place is full of Austrian prisoners, and they are turned on to do all the work. They do all the heavy work, carrying stretchers, cleaning, etc.; also we have six to clean our hospital and keep it. It sounds as

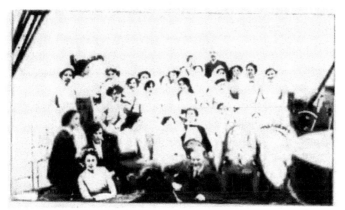

1st Serbian Unit under Dr. Eleanor Soltan

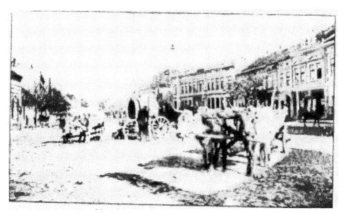

Main Street in Kraguievatz

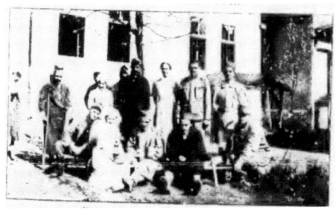

Staff and Patients, Kraguievatz

if we might be very well looked after, but they are not much good at housework.

Kraguievatz,
Thursday, 28th January 1915.

There are quite a number of hospitals in the town one of them being reserved for fever case, of which there are a great many. There is a lady doctor working there, Dr. Ross, a native of Tain. She has six wards to look after, and no nurses, only orderlies, and some times she is glad to come over here for a change. There has been no wood all day in their hospital, either for cooking or heating. She says there is always something awanting there— one day no bread, another day no eggs, or no milk. Our people have also had no wood in the hospital for two days.

The steward of a neighbouring hospital kindly offered to get supplies for us. He buys for his own hospital of 600 beds and can get us our supplies rather cheaper than I could buy them in the market or in the shops, so I go to him every afternoon with my orders. His hospital is in a school building, the gymnasium, and every day I have to pass through corridors where wounded men are lying on mattresses on the floor, as closely packed as possible, the rooms being all filled with more seriously ill. There are so many hospitals in the town that nearly all, or a very large proportion, of the men on meets are damaged in one way or another.

Things seem to be a queer mix up here. Many of the soldiers we see look like peasants in their own dress, with a rifle put into their hands, while the officers wear particularly smart uniforms. There are some very good shops here, showing very beautiful materials, probably very dear, and Parisian fashions. There is an agency of Singer Sewing Machines Co. and Coats' thread is to be got.

The language question is rather complicated. In the whole company there are three Serbian grammars, and several dictionaries, Serbian-German. Nobody has time to study seriously, so it just means that we pick up a few words as we go along. An interview with a laundress usually involves four people. The matron speaks English, the laundress Serbian, I come in with German, and the kitchen-maid with German and Serbian. The same thing has happened with other business. I have been called upon to act as interpreter for the X ray operator, who only knows a little German. At first the place was a veritable Tower of Babel. There were a few orderlies about, and when we tried to speak to them, they would shake their heads in answer, one Czech, another Magyar (all Austrian prisoners). These men were taken away and other six, German-speaking ones, arrived.

It seems that about three-fourths of the Austrian Army are Slavs, and probably sympathetic with the Serbs. Of the men we have, two are teachers, one is an official from Vienna, one a farmer, one a day labourer from the Tyrol, and the other a business porter. They have nearly all been ill since coming here, and two are away with fever. Some of them had been wounded, and all are run down with what they have come through. One is lame with frostbitten feet. They do the rough work for us. The woman who assists me is an Austrian, but was married to a Serb, and lived in Schabatz, on the Save. Her husband is missing, and she lost her home and one of her children in the bombardment of the town. On the whole they are all good friends, and between them all I have quite a nice time.

Towards the end of January the grim horrors of typhus darkened the land. On 23rd January Dr. Soltan telegraphed and wrote to the committee in Edinburgh. The telegram ran as follows:

Dire necessity for fever nurses. Can you send me ten or more overland? . . . Equipment, mattresses. Covers, blankets, linen, milk, typhol, carbolic, tow, castor-oil.'

In the letter she tells of a conference of the medical men and women working in Serbia, held at Skoplje, and gives details of her plan for opening, with the approval of the Serbian authorities, a special typhus hospital in Kraguievatz.

In answer to this letter Dr. Inglis wrote as follows:

Edinburgh, 9th March 1915.
Dear Dr. Soltan,—Thanks very much for your two interesting letters of the 23rd and 24th of February, telling of the Conference at Skoplje and of your decision to take up typhus work at Kraguievatz. I feel sure that you are perfectly right, and you may count on our support. I shall write again officially tomorrow from the Committee. I knew when you went out that we could

147

trust you to take the best line under the circumstances, and not to be bound by red tape or any conventions whatsoever, and I feel sure that your decision about the typhus hospital is right.

Your second lot of ten nurses started on Saturday with one cook. I sent you a telegram immediately after. Unfortunately, only the medical stores arrived in time to catch the transport. The rest got held up somewhere on one of the three lines of rail they had to go over between Edinburgh and Newport. I was dreadfully distressed when I heard it, because I knew how you were wanting extra sheets and blankets and all the rest of the equipment. However. Mr. Smith's letter came, saying that Sir Thomas Lipton would be able to take things out for us in the *Erin*, and we wrote to him at once asking how soon he could do this. If he will do it, and do it soon, it will probably be better than sending it by the next transport, as he will take it all the way to Salonica.

I suppose it will be quite possible to keep your surgical hospital going as well as the new typhus one! As you say, you will give your staff the choice of whether they will go there or not.

I do feel so for you having all the extra worry of these serious cases over and above the very strenuous work you have to do, and I do hope that soon we shall be able to send you out more help—indeed, I very much hope I shall be able to come myself with the next unit if we send one.—Yours very sincerely,

Elsie Maud Inglis.

Kraguievatz, 13th February 1915.[2]

As for us, we are quite settled down, and seem to have been here for months. The hospital is set going now, and I believe we have under our supervision about 300 patients, which, of course, is three times the number we were prepared to have, but which is a miserably small number out of the thousands of patients that there are, even in this town alone. We have a school and another building attached, and four small "*gast* houses" for the more convalescent cases. The other hospitals are so badly off for accommodation, beds, clothes and comforts of any description, that the comfort of our place seems almost selfish luxury. I have never seen anything like the places we have seen since we came here

---

2. The story of the hospital continued.

The hospitals here are just like those at Nish only they are not quite so closely packed. The patients are lying mostly on straw mattresses on the floor, or on wooden beds with only a rug over them, and often only the clothes which they had on in the battlefield. Their food which consists of hard black bread always, and sometimes meat or eggs, etc., lies beside them, also the few earthly belongings which they have managed to keep by them.

There has been an outbreak of enteric fever in the trenches, and the patients are coming in every day in bullock-carts from the north, and the authorities are clearing as many patients out of the hospitals as they can to make room for them. Until the conditions can be changed in the hospitals, I am afraid the outlook for the patients is pretty hopeless, but it seems to me the Serbs have been overwhelmed with the numbers of sick and wounded, and scarcely know how to tackle things

Our hospital makes a very bright spot in the midst of it all, but we seem to be able to do so little compared with the amount there is to be done. We have already wired home for more nurses and doctors at the instigation of the Serbian Government. and are hoping that we may ultimately be able to do something on a larger scale. We have just heard that the British Red Cross Society are coming out with doctors and nurses, and are to stay in the house across the way from us, so altogether there will be quite a large British contingent among us. Our patients are enjoying. and thriving in, the comfort we have been able to give them. It was a great pleasure to see the joy they had in being clean in a clean bed.

Most of them have horribly septic wounds, which through pressure of work are only being dressed every four or five days. They are nearly all young men about twenty or twenty-five, but some of them look like fifty. We are gradually restoring their youth to some of them. When they are ill, they are very patient, and when they are well, they are lively and happy. I am sorry to say they just get well to be sent back to the ranks again. The Serbs are certainly a magnificent race of men, and live simple, good lives, and would be happy if they had not to fight. We spend most of the day doing dressings, either in the dressing-rooms or in the wards.

We have an x-ray apparatus fitted up in the house we use as

the home, and have to carry the patients along on stretchers to be x-rayed. One night we had been busy examining patients, and had taken our current from the main which supplies only the crown prince's house and the x-ray outfit. Next morning an official was sent along to request that we do all the x-raying before a stated hour, as the night before the crown prince had been left in complete darkness!

We have a very happy time in the home. Last night was full moon and hard frost, so three of us set out for a walk in the snow. It was quite exquisite, and we got out into the country, and had a good tramp. I have never felt the cold so keenly, and today my cheeks are quite burnt with the sting.

In March, to Dr, Soltan's everlasting credit, she added to the work of her surgical hospital, which was full of patients, the complete charge of a hospital for typhus cases, a burden which was gladly undertaken by her already hard-worked staff.

The hospital[3] was quite half a mile from our home lying as it did on the outskirts of the town, but we were generally glad of the walk, and attributed partly to it that the health of the nurses remained so good. Certainly after rain a few remarks have been made about Serbian roads in general, and this one in particular, for the mud was thick and deep, and ponds were many. In the evenings, coming home, it was quite dark, and often rainy, but a little *fainijer* (lantern) guided our steps, and our hearts were light with the knowledge of good work being done. Two sentries guarded the entrance to the road which led on to the hospital, and always the *Englesha Sestra* were cordially greeted with *Dobro utro!* (Good morning), and *Laku notch!* (Goodnight).

Our costume in the wards was hardly that of the stereotyped English nurse, with a cap and apron and stiff collar, and our friends would not have recognised us, but precautions have to be taken to prevent infection. Instead of the usual uniform and apron, we wore a white cotton combination garment, with the ends tucked into high leather riding boots. Over this, for the sake of appearance, an overall was worn, and our hair was entirely covered with a tight-fitting cap. Round neck and arms we wore bandages soaked in camphor oil, and our boots were smeared with the same, so that no encouragement was given to

---

3. By a sister in the fever hospital.

the little insect by which typhus is spread.

We met with all sorts of typhus complications, but how good it was to see men recover whose cases seemed so hopeless at first! Serbian men make splendid patients. For the most part, they do as they are told, and take their medicine very obediently—an excellent thing in patients—but if at any time a man, perhaps delirious or newly submitted, was inclined to talk at medicine or nourishment, there was sure to be hand some convalescent ready to explain how the medicine the *Sestra* had given him had made him better. They were so like children, these big men, that we could not help getting very fond of our patients, and certainly we were more than repaid by their gratitude.

It is only fair to say, that we were greatly helped in the wards by our orderlies, for the most part Austrian prisoners, between whom and the patients there existed a wonderfully good feeling. Among our patients were occasional prisoners, but they were treated just the same by orderlies and patients alike, and frequently it was only when a man was convalescent that we discovered him to be a prisoner. The Serbs bear their enemies no ill-will.

We found it necessary to open a women's ward—one day without any warning, a woman was brought and left with us—and it was greatly appreciated. We had our share of babies who accompanied their mothers, and who were, of course, great pets. One little Zygani baby, a little dark beauty, was in great demand in the men's wards, for above everything these great, big, strong Serbian men love children, and they are very fond of flowers. Underneath their practical exterior lies a deep vein of poetry, and they are lovers of music and the open country. Plucky they are to a degree, and unafraid of death—perhaps because they have so often met it face to face.

Later still, a third hospital for recurrent fever was taken over in the town. By the end of March the Scottish Women were responsible for 550 beds. For the hospital for recurrent fever only one doctor could be spared, but it was wonderful what these two women accomplished.

Dreadful as was the state of things in Kraguievatz, news kept coming of a much worse condition of affairs in Valjevo, a little town farther north. There the wounded and fever-stricken men lay in their uniforms, absolutely untended.

After her return home Dr. Soltan told the committee how incessantly Valjevo had been on her heart but how impossible it had been for her to organise any help for the sufferers. Then she added:

> Though I could not get up to Valjevo, one day Valjevo came down to me. A row of bullock-carts drew up at the hospital gates one morning—they were laden with men from Valjevo.

It was impossible to refuse them. They were taken in, and though the ordinary work of the hospital went on as usual, the necessary operations were performed on these men. Every one was suffering from gangrenous wounds. The work was overwhelming. Dr. Soltan contracted diphtheria, and the chief surgeon being also laid aside with typhus, Dr. Soltan wired for Dr. Inglis. It was to this hospital that Dr Inglis came out in May 1915 The "long-drawn-out battle" was drawing to a close when she landed in Serbia. Help had been sent from nearly every country in Europe, and Serbia "was fast becoming the cleanest country on earth." The dread disease had taken terrible toll of those who had fought so valiantly against it. It did not spare, too, the staff, of the Scottish Women's Hospital: three out of the fifty who had been sent out during these tragic months laid down their lives—Sister Jordan, Miss Madge Neil Fraser, and Sister Minshull.

On 11th May Dr. Inglis sent home to the committee her first report from Serbia, part of which is given:

Report from Dr. Elsie Inglis

The unit here is in charge of three hospitals, Reserve No. 3 (surgical), Reserve No. 6 (typhus), and Reserve No. 7 (relapsing fever), and a considerable amount of phthisis and general disease). The important department of No. 7 is the Receiving Room, where the patients have to be diagnosed and distributed to the other hospitals: especially is it of importance just now, because of the typhus epidemic.

The Surgical Hospital, No. 3. Is in the town, a schoolhouse in two blocks, with a long courtyard between them. Down one side is a covered shed, part of which is used as a kitchen for the patients, part as a laundry, part for the Austrian orderlies to sleep in, and the rest as a place for the convalescent patients to sit in. The hospital holds 170 beds, and is at present nearly full. Mostly convalescents or old bad cases, but a certain number of surgical cases continue to come in. There are a great many cases for daily dressings. Both the operating theatre and the room for the dressings are beautifully arranged and managed by Sister Boykett and are very creditable to an improvised hospital.

The wards are small, and there are too many beds in each, according to our standards, but many fewer than there are in other hospitals I have seen here. The wards are quite fresh: the windows always open.

The hospital is at present under the charge of Dr. Chesney, who is doing excellent work. It is understaffed as regards sisters, most of them having been drafted over to the Typhus Hospital. The five nurses being sent on by Dr. Hutchison from Malta (who we chosen for this unit) arrive tonight, and matron intends to arrange that there are two night sisters, one in each block, four day sisters, two in each block

The Typhus hospital, No. 6, is on the outskirts of the town, a big square building, which was I believe, barracks. It holds 200 patients, is overcrowded, from our standard, but is clean and fresh and well arranged. It is comparatively well staffed, fourteen sisters, and when the new ones arrive, sixteen. But its equipment might be immensely unproved. The doctors who are working there are—Dr. M'Vea, Dr. Corbett, and Dr. Laird.

The Relapsing Fever Hospital, No. 7. This is in a building quite near No. 6, in the open county (the real objection to both is that they stand on low ground). It was an old palace, and then barracks, which had been condemned. It was empty when it was turned into a hospital. It is in two storeys. A long corridor runs the whole length of the building, both upstairs and down. Off them open the rooms, downstairs the patients are received, upstairs are the wards, comparatively small square rooms; all overcrowded. The place will hold 200 beds, and has now 170 patients. The kitchen and laundry are outside.

It has no equipment to speak of, and is being worked by Dr. Brooke and one sister, namely. Sister Hollway! This, of course, sounds ridiculous, and it is so in a sense. There is very little nursing or doctoring. But there is no denying that those two women have worked wonders in the place. The Austrian orderlies are kept up to their duties. The patients, at any rate, get the medicines which are ordered for them, and the place is fairly clean.

For the present, until the committee can send out more nurses, the best we can do is to put on another day sister (so that the

153

two on day duty may be able to get proper time off), and a night sister. At present Sister Hollway goes on duty at seven, and stays on till five except for dinner, and Dr. Brooke makes her evening visit between six and seven, and after that the Austrian orderlies are left with no supervision.

This is the work the unit *has undertaken*. It means that they made themselves responsible, for something like 570 beds! One can quite understand how they were almost driven into it, in the face of the awful country, and there is no doubt at all that they have done it excellently, and with a wonderful self-devotion. The standard in all three hospitals is distinctly higher than that of the ordinary hospital here, and the Surgical Hospital is really well equipped and well arranged. The Serbian Consul at Salonika told us that General Soubitich, the Chief Medical Officer of the Serbian Army, had told him that the Scottish Women's Hospital was the best in Serbia; and the consul added that one thing that had made their work so helpful was that they did not 'expect impossibilities of the country,' but made the best of what they could get.

I have heard the same thing several times, and Mr. Des Graz, the British Minister at Nish, told me that he could not speak too, highly of the splendid work that had been done.

The Scottish Women were the second unit to reach Serbia in its time of need. Lady Paget with her hospital had the proud distinction of being the first. She was in the country as early as October 1914, and her hospital at Skoplje did magnificent work through the typhus epidemic and the "long, peaceful summer." She remained at her post after the Bulgar occupation of the town, where she was taken prisoner, and did not reach England again until March 1916. She was decorated by the Crown Prince of Serbia with the order of St. Sava, First Class, a cross of diamonds.

In a letter to Lady Brassey in August 1915, Lady Paget says of the S.W.H.:

The Scottish Women's Units are doing splendid work all over the country, and are much appreciated by the Serbians, and what makes them especially valuable to this country is their adaptability. They are ready and willing to adapt themselves to any condition or circumstances; they never grumble or complain, are always cheerful and smiling, always ready to lend a helping hand to any British or Serbian Unit who are hard pressed. And their courage and the way they overcome almost insurmountable difficulties is extraordinary. Ralph and the Serbians have nothing but praise of them, and if all your nurses are like the three we have here, then they must indeed be gems. [4] I must say I think great credit is due to your 'Selecting Committee' for the way they choose their staff, for I have rarely come across a nicer lot of people than those in the S. W. Units. People speak very highly of the qualifications of Mrs. Haverfield as an organiser and administrator. I hear she is extraordinarily capable and hard working and energetic. Of all the units out here the S.W.H. have done the best work, so the committee need not feel it has wasted its money.

From among the many stories of our patients we give one full of pathos:

Another boy, a real Austrian, had been shot in the head, and had a certain part of his brain destroyed, so that he is quite blind. He cried bitterly when Dr. Hollway asked him, how long he had been so. When he had been put to bed we asked him if he needed anything, and he asked for the loaf of bread he had brought with him, and sat up and ate it like a wolf. We asked if he felt better, and he said, '*Ja, ich geh,*' quite tonelessly. Mostly he lies without a sound. I pray he may die.

I visited the blind Austrian boy who is in Sister Hollway's ward where Miss Shepherd is 'Pro,' just to offer him 'New Year' greetings. He asked us whether the war was still going on. I suppose the poor child has been lying among foreigners for weeks. We told him we were from Scotland, and he confided in us. He asked to be helped to write to his sister, his only relative. He has no idea of how long he has been blind and a prisoner. . . . We are getting one of the house orderlies who is our '*tablemaitre*' and an ex-schoolmaster to see him tomorrow, and write his letter for him. I cannot imagine anything more awful than that boy has been through, that feeling of being blind and helpless and utterly lost among his enemies. Poor little Samson. Worse because he knows only his own language. . . .

On Friday we brought the *lehrer* to visit our Austrian boy, and they had a very long conversation together, during which the

---

4. Three of the Scottish Women were lent to Lady Paget at this time.

155

letter was written. It was handed over to a Serbian Red Cross major afterwards and will get through, I believe. . . .

This morning, Saturday, our Austrian boy Johann found to his delight that his sight had partly returned. He could make out my head and shoulders quite quickly. The *lehrer* was delighted at his news, and told me that poor Johann had asked *der liebe Gott* that he might see again. . . . .

Our x-ray apparatus now works very well and Dr. McDougal is quite in the best circles of Serbian society, we tell her, for officers come to her, even from Nish. We had several of Dr. Hollway's cases today, including Johann Frenzel, the half-blind boy. He can see better every day, he says, and now can make out some colours, but cannot tell one person from another. I pay him a call every evening; he is really a very interesting case. He has been moved into another of Sister Hollway's wards, where the patients are very kind to him. He is getting over his nervous breakdown, thanks very largely I think to Miss Shepherd, *die kleine schwester*, who is so patient with him, and another Serbian boy, who is really hardly human and is always crying out. Poor Johann gives no trouble like this, he was only too resigned at first, but he is getting better.

It is a relief to leave Johann restored to sight and friends. If the Scottish Women had done no more than save this poor laddie from darkness and loneliness those who sent them out would have felt it had been worthwhile. But multiply Johann ten thousandfold and you get nearer the number of those who have been healed and helped and made happy by the members of the S.W.H.

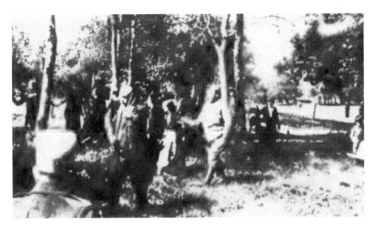

SERBIAN FETE DAY

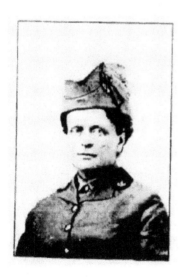

DR. INGLIS IN SERBIA

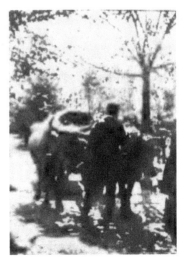

BREAD CART

CHAPTER 3

"The Long, Peaceful Summer"

The story of the summer of 1915, between the two storms of the typhus epidemic and the invasion by the enemy, is told in the following chapter in Dr. Inglis' own words. The quotations are taken from her weekly letters to the committee. We see in them how the work of the S.W.H. grew during those months, and they bring Dr. Inglis before us vividly Her extraordinary genius for organising (shared in by so many of the women who have worked in the units) makes itself felt; and in her description of visits of inspection to the hospitals and camps of the S.W H and of her many journeys, from one town to another, to interview the necessary authorities for the furtherance of her many schemes, her energetic spirit lives before us. The letters are full of numerous references to her beloved Serbs, and readers will be glad to know that "the lost *Gloucester Castle* equipment," so often mentioned, and for which such untiring search was made, was eventually found.

"The peaceful summer" contains the story of the Valjevo Unit. This, the 3rd Unit of the S.W.H. left England in April under Dr. Alice Hutchison. It was detained at Malta a fortnight by Lord Methuen to look after our British wounded, and then on arrival in Serbia was sent to Valjevo—"poor little Valjevo," which had been so much on Dr. Soltan's heart. The equipment for this hospital was the finest yet sent out by the S.W.H. Extracts from Dr. Hutchison's letters given at the end of this chapter describe the work of the unit at Malta and at Valjevo.

When Dr. Inglis arrived in Serbia the idea of those in authority was to have a line of "blocking hospitals" in the north—at Mladanovatz, Posheravatz, and Palanka. These hospitals were to act as disinfecting camps, preventing any infectious diseases brought by the army from spreading again into Serbia. The surgical cases only were to be

158

brought down to Kraguievatz. The Scottish Women's Hospitals were to provide these three camps. Dr. Hutchison's Unit, which was then on its way from home, "the finest hospital under canvas ever sent to the Balkans," was to be sent to Posheravatz. Of the three hospitals at Kraguievatz the two fever ones were to be closed, and the staff, with their equipment supplemented by Sir Ralph Paget from his store, were to form one Camp Hospital at Mladanovatz; for the Palanka Camp reinforcements were wired for from Scotland.

Eventually this scheme fell through, but the S.W.H. formed a line in the north, though not exactly in the same formation as had been planned. Their blocking line was composed of the two camp hospitals at Valjevo and Mladanovatz, under Drs. Hutchison and McGregor respectively, and a Serbian hospital at Lazarovatz staffed by the Scottish Women under Dr. Hollway.

DR. INGLIS' LETTERS.

Nish, 4th June 1915.

What brought me up to Nish was to see Sir Ralph Paget about the new scheme, and also Dr. Hutchison. Her unit had been stopped here, because a bridge has come down in the floods north of Kraguievatz and south of Posheravatz, Dr Hutchison's equipment is, however, south of the bridge, and it has been suddenly decided by the Serbian authorities that she is to go to Valjevo at once, as the bridge cannot be mended for ten days. Of course she is delighted, as that means work at once; but it knocks the 'scheme,' which was a very much bigger thing,— and I am safe in saying Colonel Hunter's idea,—on the head. The scheme was to block the whole infectious disease, which always appears in every army, up north, by these three big disinfecting camps, and to bring only surgical cases south of Kraguievatz. Now we again begin simply attacks on isolated centres like Valjevo, which from all accounts is bad enough, but unless we can make Mladanovatz very fine and effective, I am afraid whatever attacks the army will attack Serbia—as typhus did. I am writing; quite frankly, as this letter is to be brought by hand.

Dr. Hutchison is looking very well, and all her unit whom I have seen—very pleased, too, with what they were able to do at Malta. Sir Ralph say the governor has written him a most eulogistic letter. I wonder if the War Office would let us send a real unit for our own men there. . . .

You can think of us really being of use—all three hospitals at Kraguievatz have been full and very busy. In the surgical one last week we had twenty-three operations, and one man told Dr. Chesney that he was going to write to his brother—a doctor in Bosnia (he is a prisoner)—what magnificent surgeons the English are. Major Protitch says this is the 'best surgical hospital in Serbia,' but you must not take that too literally: they are awfully kind people, and love saying pleasant things. Did I ever tell you that our doctor's uniform hat is really the Serbian Army hat? I was amused when I first saw it.

Kraguievatz, 10th June 1915.

And now for our news. My last letter went from Nish taken by Captain Bennett, and I told you Dr. Hutchison had been ordered to Valjevo. Sir Ralph got Colonel Hunter to come up. and everything seemed all right, and we arranged that she and her sanitary inspector and her three men should come on that night with me, and the unit follow in two days. Suddenly—at six o'clock in the evening—she got orders to take her whole unit up at once. The train started at eight. With great good luck she collected them all, and even fed them, except two who were found missing at the station, and Dr. Phillips had to go back for them. These sudden bursts of energy in a people who generally love delay are terribly upsetting!

One delightful Serbian officer—at Mladanovatz, where I spent a weary hour trying to nail Colonel —— down to which site he intended to give us for our camp—suddenly leaned forward and said to me in English 'Don't lose heart, Madam: things go slower in Serbia than in England!' I did laugh. I might have said to him that there are cataclysms in Serbia which break the slow monotony, and certainly one of them carried Dr Hutchison s Unit up to Valjevo. There is another funny thing about Serbia, and that is that you seldom get the reason for anything. I told you that Dr. Hutchison's Unit could not go to Posheravatz because a bridge was down. Well! will you believe it, there was no bridge down?

The next morning at Lapobo. the junction at 3 a.m. we found Mrs. Haverfield, Mr. Smith, and Colonel Michalovitz, and when we all exclaimed. 'How did you get here?' they said that there was no railway bridge down at all, only a road bridge which did not affect the traffic. So why Dr. Hutchison went to Valjevo remains a mystery. It *may* have been because there were movements of troops near the frontier at Posheravatz; it *may* have been because Miss Christitch has arrived at Valjevo, and wants a hospital. Anyhow, it was *not* a broken bridge, and she is at a point there where she is much needed, and she is by now fully installed. . . .

. . . She leaned out of the window that morning, on the train, with all her pretty red hair fluffy, in a blue *kimono*. I was dreadfully afraid all these people I introduced her to would not realise she was really head of a unit! However, I know that would not long after they had had dealings with her.

And now about our camp al Mladanovatz. After innumerable delays, finally Mrs. Haverfield, Dr. Laird (who is, I told you, to stay here permanently in the Surgical Hospital), and I went off in Colonel Gentitch's car, with him and another Serbian officer, to Mladanovatz for the wildest motor drive I ever had in my life. We skidded at least fifty times in the course of the day, but we never upset. We bumped all the day, and at one time charged a string of boulders, which had been used to mend the road, and, and *got over them*: but it was the most glorious run as regards scenery.

For a long way the road ran along the top of hills, and we had the most wonderful distant views of hills and valleys, and the lights and shadows were magnificent. I don't know when I enjoyed anything so much. And we did the business we set out to do, namely, chose our site. Unfortunately Colonel Michalovitz was still at Valjevo, and Colonel Hunter had just got his orders to go straight off to Malta, and could not spare the time to come; but one of his men. Captain C——, was there, and came up in the nick of time; so we got a very good site, gently sloping ground, with a good water-supply, and an iron shed at the back where we can put stores. . . .

We shall miss Colonel Hunter and his young men very much. They have been extraordinarily helpful. Tomorrow the equipment goes. Matron and Sister Brown have done all the separating and packing beautifully. Sir Ralph Paget gave me 300 sheets and with these and your most generous equipment we can keep the Surgical Hospital here fully up to the mark, and manage 300 beds at Mladanovatz.

Mladanovatz, 16th June 1915.
The camp is on a slope facing the s.w., and there is the most glorious view you can imagine across the valley, and away to high hills in the distance. It has been hard but most interesting work getting the hospital arranged, but now we are practically ready, and patients may come any day—indeed we expected some today. . . . .

I wish you could see our kitchen—the quaintest little place, in a shed, which was here when we came, and to which we have added another shed, the whole open all round. *And* our incinerator—which I built! It burns up everything so beautifully!"

The part of the letter which follows refers to a question that had arisen. As the country was now comparatively free of disease, were the S.W.H. and other hospital units to accept this as likely to be a permanent condition, and withdraw from Serbia to centres of greater need, or was provision to be made for the treatment of the wounded from the battles which would follow the arrival of the British and French forces then confidently expected? It will be seen what decision was arrived at, at a conference of the various hospital units held later.

As to the future development of the work, your telegram came this morning asking if the Serbian authorities and Sir Ralph Paget want another unit here, and it was that that finally decided me to go back morrow and see the Chief of the Medical Department, Colonel Gentitch. There is no doubt that there is very little sickness in the country at present. The whole point is how much they mean to prepare for the future and I'll wire after I have seen him. The last two letters I have written will explain the situation, so I need not go into it again. Mrs. Hunter's letter has arrived in which she says the committee propose rather to strengthen and equip the units already out than send new ones; and that is an excellent policy at present.

Our director here is very nice—Dr. Zdravkovitch—most anxious to help in every way. He is in charge of another camp, a little nearer the village, on the same hill. A trench marks the boundary between the camps, and they call it 'the Straits of Dover'! We messed with them at first, but now we have our own kitchen in working order, and all our unit is up here.

I got a *Scotsman* yesterday showing that the funds have reached £28,000—apparently apart from the Welsh and London funds. *Good!* What about a unit to Malta, or Alexandria, for our own men? Lord Methuen would welcome them! He was very loath to let Dr Hutchison's Unit come away.

Kraguievatz, 22nd June 1915.

The Valjevo camp is beautifully situated, lower down the valley than that at Mladanovatz, but on sloping ground with a good water-supply. It is, of course thoroughly well arranged, and every detail well thought out, as you would expect from Dr. Hutchison. General M——, the general in command of the Drina district came to see it when I was there, and was very pleased with the whole thing. (Mladanovatz is under the Belgrade command.)

Wood is very precious here, so we have decided at Mladanovatz not to put down our wooden-floors, but to use the planks for dividing up the magazine. That would have cost us £40 otherwise. The only tent in which we will put a wooden floor is the operating theatre, and there we shall make it in four pieces. There will be no heavy beds, and we shall empty the theatre once a week, take out the floor and scrub it, and spray the ground with formalin.

In the other tents we have cleared away the thick grass, beaten the ground hard, and dug a deep trench round to carry off the rain-water. The ground in the tents is sprayed with formalin every morning.

There were seventy patients in yesterday morning at Mladanovatz when I left, and they are coming in at the rate of fifteen to twenty a day—medical cases entirely. Some of them seem to be cases of pure fatigue. They arrive with a temperature of 103° or 104°, they are put to bed, given milk and some light supper, and the next morning the temperature is normal. Then after a day or two they begin to rouse up. There were two bad pneumonias in, a case of rheumatic fever, and a man who might possibly be enteric. Everybody is settling down splendidly to their work. . . .

. . . One day I got a message from Colonel Gentitch to say he would like to come over to say goodbye to the staff, who were going to Mladanovatz, and see some Scottish dances, after dinner. So I at once wrote off and asked him to come to dinner; and I also asked Captain Javanovitch—the censor—and Dr. Kopje, and Colonel Harrison, and we had a very nice evening. Two nights after, they gave a banquet to the departing unit which I missed, having started for Mladanovatz; and he made the most extraordinarily warm speech, in which he said the Scottish Women's Units were always first in the field, first when the war broke out, and first when the bombs fell.

But perhaps the thing that will interest the committee most was a conversation I had with Dr. Curcin. He said to me that he did hope we would not lose patience, and that we would realise that one of the greatest difficulties in Serbia is that they are not used to women doing this sort of work. He said, 'At the bottom of his heart Colonel —— can never believe that a woman can do a thing as well as a man! And,' he said, 'the most of the men in Serbia are like that! Now I know,' he said, ' that that is absurd, and, Madam, I want you to realise that I, and the men who think like me, the advanced party, we are almost more grateful to you for coming out and showing what women can do, than for the hospitals you have given us.'—Now, wasn't that nice?

As regards the work out here, when the move comes, and I suppose that will be when Constantinople falls, or the Russians gain a decisive victory, there will be a tremendous need for us! The whole army is massed on the frontier, a quarter of a million of men (I am offending the censor, so you will be careful—won't you?). We see them streaming past at Mladanovatz, and they have only about 300 Serbian doctors altogether. One hundred and twenty-five of their doctors died during the typhus outbreak; so you will see how short-handed they must be. And we all know now how long it takes to get out help from home, therefore it seems to me that the help ought to be *ready*.

. . . . By the way, Mrs. Hunter says you have been criticised for the meagreness of your equipment. *What* things people will say! Why, we are running 450 beds at this moment with an equipment you sent out for 300! And with only sheets and towels for 100 beds we shall run 550 beds *easily! And* in two hospitals—which means the duplication of many things.

Sir Ralph Paget has given us some delightful boxes of stores. P.S.—just home from the conference at Mrs Stobart's. General Soubititch. Head of the Red Cross, was there and Captain Javanovitch. There is no uncertainty about it at all. Colonel Gentitch said definitely that *no one is to leave*, and all units on the way *to come at once*. Captain Javanovitch put it that this is 'the lull before the storm.' It is reported today that the German emperor has invited the Prime Ministers of Bulgaria and Roumania to visit him at his headquarters. If they go against us there will be savage fighting here. Then there is a possibility that Germany may try to break through to help the Turks in the Dardanelles. In any case 'there is a storm brewing, and we must have everything taut for the gale.' They did not mince matters at all. and I pass it all on to you, knowing that you will remember that the *censor has not seen this letter.*

Kraguievatz 1st July 1915.
I only wish you could see both camps at Valjevo and Mladanovatz. They are both in perfectly lovely country and well placed. It was curious to go up on the hill the evening I was with Dr. Hutchison, and look down on that peaceful valley, and the clean little white town and think what a change had come there since the winter.

With Miss Holme arrived the two motors—the Welsh ambulance and the seven-seater. Will you tell the donors how very pleased we were to see them, and how much they have been admired, especially the Welsh ambulance, which we have been told is the finest ambulance in Serbia. I cannot say I *hope* they will soon be in use, but I can say this, if the need arises, which is expected, it is a great thing to have two such cars ready Sir Ralph Paget says he will lend us two other ambulances in that contingency also, till our other ones come out.

Everything depends so much on events over which we have no control, and there are so many possible contingencies that it is very difficult to say definitely what should be done, to my mind, but this much is certain that if anything does happen, this plucky little country will need help more than any other of our Allies, and we have definitely undertaken to help them.

One way and another I have been able to see a good deal of the country going from one of our hospitals to another, and up to Belgrade, and so on. Most people find the travelling very tiring, but I must say I have enjoyed it all. I have had the most extraordinary luck—the government have given me a free pass over all the railways. Once I got into a Sanitary train and was invited to breakfast by one of the doctors in charge. I generally find my travelling companions most interesting and ready to talk: I have travelled with Serbian officers, who have told me a lot about the country.

I am going to take this letter down to the censor tomorrow and if he passes it I shall register it home. I don't know that I have thrown much light on your problem. You must know better than we out here do where most help is needed, and perhaps events will have settled the question before this letter arrives. Anyhow, we have all our plans ready, and my own feeling is that we can probably be more helpful here than anywhere, though I *would* like a hospital ship at the Dardanelles

Kraguievatz 10th July 1915.

I have just been reading an article in the *Times* which gives a very good account of the conditions here now. You have probably seen it. The typhus is over, there is no fighting for the moment, and the country is wonderfully healthy. Sir Ralph Paget is coming to Kraguievatz tomorrow—and has summoned a conference of the heads of British Units to consider the position. I shall finish this letter tomorrow after the conference and tell you what takes place. My own feeling strongly is that we should wait here in readiness for emergencies *which must come*, and when they come there will be no country in more need than Serbia—with under 300 doctors and no nurses whatsoever. In the meantime, it seems to me there is a good deal we can do here. As soon as our drugs arrive, and our tent-poles—which have stuck for some unknown reason in Salonique—Dr. McGregor is going to open a dispensary for the civil population at Mladanovatz.

Then we are arranging for Dr. Hollway and the new doctors, with some sisters, to take over a Serbian hospital at Lazarovatz, and run it.

...We are waiting to hear from Lazarovatz. And I think it ought to be a most interesting bit of work, and also a very fine experiment. I should like to see what could be made of a Serbian hospital, using their own workmen and their own things, and see how much more is really needed. And Dr. Hollway likes the Serbians so much that it ought to work out well. In a small way,

I have been trying the same in our Surgical Hospitals here—for the new theatre and the improved sanitary arrangements, etc. In the theatre, for instance, instead of taking the glass cupboard for instruments, which we might have had from the things sent out by the British Government to Colonel Hunter, I have had a first-rate wooden cupboard made by an ordinary carpenter, and painted white. And the iron stands, for the lotion bowls, Colonel Darrach is making for us at the Arsenal. And it is going to be as nice a theatre as any in Serbia.

By the way, I got the concrete floor after all, thanks to Lieutenant R——, the engineer officer who is carrying out our improvements. Getting the courtyard in order has been quite exciting work. The cesspool, they admit, has not been emptied for four years. I think it is more like ten. We have pumped and pumped, and then last night they tried to empty it with buckets. One of the carts broke down and upset the whole awful mess in the street. It was perfectly awful. We have been at it for five mortal weeks. We have done, however, more in three days than we managed the three weeks before.

They sent down ten Austrians to fill in a dreadful pit of dirty water, but they sent no picks or shovels! There were exactly two shovels and one pick in hospital, and when I went down eight Austrians were lying under the trees smoking—two were leisurely throwing loose earth into the pit. When they got to the end, another man dragged himself to his feet and broke up some more ground with the pick while the two overworked shovellers smoked. I watched this for about ten minutes, and then I descended on them. I asked for the officer in charge; they said there wasn't one. Ten Austrian prisoners and nobody in charge you know!!

Eventually we found the Serbian non-commissioned officer *asleep* at the back of the bathroom. I stood over them for two hours, and I don't think those Austrians can have worked so hard since they came to Serbia. They worked in five-minute shifts three at a time, one breaking up earth and the other two shovelling. In two hours we had made the slope where the cart is to stand which is to carry away our dirty water, and thrown all the earth into the pit. Then I went up to Colonel G——'s office and said that if they wanted me to spend my time standing over Austrian orderlies I was quite willing to do it, but I thought it was a job for their officers.

They were horrified. So all yesterday and today there has been feverish energy, and the place is tidied out of knowledge. We have half (!) emptied the cesspool. We have built an incinerator for all the dressings (which before went into the pond!) and solid refuse from the kitchen. We made a '*tamp*,' namely, a slope in which a cart with two barrels will stand, and all dirty water will be emptied into them, and carted to the fields. We are to have two carts and a yoke of oxen, but don't be surprised if you find I have bought a yoke of oxen for you, for we shall find it much easier to keep our carts circulating if we control them entirely.

And we have filled in the awful pit or pond—*and* the Serbians have tidied up the grass, which is so like them, the dear things. While we struggle with the cesspool they make the grass nice.

Well, that hospital will be a demonstration in Kraguievatz of what they can or ought to do on their own system with their own implements. Everybody who has seen the incinerator is so taken with it, from Colonel Gentitch, who came especially to inspect it, to the little peasant woman next door, who stood rapt in admiration saying, '*Dobra*' (good).

The conference is over. Sir Ralph and Lady Paget arrived here at 7 o'clock for breakfast, and we had the conference in our dining-room at 10 30, and half the people stayed to lunch, and everybody came back to tea and Miss Patrick's Scotch scones! The resolution, which was unanimously passed, ran as follows:

> That in view of the possibilities of the situation this conference decides that no British Unit at present in Serbia shall leave the country. The conference shall meet again in September.

It appeared that, counting the two doctors and nineteen nurses just coming to us, we are only 270 strong.

Kraguievatz, 19th July 1915.

. . . . . The Serbs are a strikingly handsome race. Our patients are delightful. The other day Dr. Chesney got up a gymkhana for them in the hospital yard—a very simple affair and they did enjoy it so. A good many of the things had to be done by the Austrian orderlies—for instance, a stretcher race, where I thought it distinctly safer to have a well man in the stretcher. But there were several events for the patients: an egg-and-spoon race, and a crutch race, and a needle-threading race—when the sisters threaded the needles. I went into the wards in the middle to give some tobacco to the men who could not come out. and heard the laughter and cheers and I could not help thinking, there we all were—Turks and British and Serbs and Austrians. all playing together as happy as possible. Perhaps if we played more together, and knew one another better, such awful things as this war would not happen. We give some simple prizes—tobacco and cigarettes and knives.

Major Protege, our director, came and said the men were obviously so well that he was going to send them back on command at once—a joke that was hugely enjoyed. Dr. Chesney organised the whole affair splendidly, and deserves a lot of credit. Somebody said to me that it had been so nice that it was a pity we had not asked if the crown prince would come and give the prizes. Of course we never thought of soaring so high; but I said I only wished I had thought of it, for then the crown prince would have noticed the awful smells in our yard, and perhaps something would have been done. However, I gave the prizes, and we ended by playing the National Anthem on the violin, and singing 'God Save the King.'....

I wish you could have seen us last Sunday afternoon. That was one of the unexpected things that happen. We went up, some of us, quite unsuspecting, on a quiet, sunshiny afternoon to the Stobart Camp for service (by the way, we have one here every Sunday), and instead of a calm service we spent the afternoon hanging on to tent-ropes and rescuing patients from under collapsed tents. The wind suddenly got up, and in about two minutes a peaceful camp was a roaring chaos. Eventually, when it died down, there were seventeen tents down, and five centre poles broken. I wish I had time to tell you of all the funny things that happened.

Almost everybody's hair came down. One patient with a crutch hurled himself out of the tent, and twisted himself and his crutch into a rope and sat down on it. In another place the patients were all found sitting in a row—on the fly—but I must say they saved the tent. Mrs. Stobart took it awfully well, and as nobody is any the worse we can all laugh as much as we like. I was so stiff I could hardly move the next day. *The* achievement was the cooks'. When we eventually emerged with time to look round, we found the kitchen fire still alight, and the evening meal being cooked, though all the tents, kitchen stores, etc.. were down. I am not sure that Mrs. Stobart did not nearly equal them, for she invited us all to stay to supper! But we didn't. . . .

I do not think you should alter the uniforms, for everybody is beginning to know it—here, at any rate—and people come up to one and say, 'You are the Scottish Women, aren't you? I travelled with your people on such and such a boat, or met them in such and such a such a place.' But could not a felt hat—soft—be added for undress uniform, exactly to match the grey of the winter uniforms? Dr. Hutchison was asking what has become of the 'serpents' for her unit?

It was nice getting a glimpse of her when she came down for the conference, looking so well. I have heard all sorts of complimentary things about her camp: its splendid sanitary arrangements and good order.

Skoplje, 10th August 1915.

The committee will be surprised at this address. Lady Paget wired to me last Sunday and again on Monday, asking me to come down and help them, as they had some bad surgical cases and no surgeon. I had already lent her three of the new sisters, and said that Dr. Hollway could come for ten days or so. Dr. Hollway was at Lazarovatz investigating the position there, and she followed me here and took over Dr. Morrison's work—he is going home next week; Mrs. Laurie knows him—125 beds and the surgical work, and he went up to Belgrade to see what he could arrange there about a surgeon. He wires that he is coming back tomorrow morning, bringing a surgeon with him. We all exclaimed, 'Well done!' So I shall go off tomorrow night—straight to Mladanovatz. and from there to Valjevo, where they are in great trouble—six cases of enteric three doctors and three sisters.

After Valjevo I shall go to Lazarovatz—which lies between Valjevo and Mladanovatz—and see them fairly started. Dr. Hollway's account is very interesting. It is a village, and the 'Hospital.' which consists of 200 beds, is in eight different houses really miscalled 'gast houses.' it is a junction, and will be a splendid dressing-station some day. We shall go thoroughly into the equipment, but Dr. Hollway says There are 1000 sheets; which makes me think they expect developments there. (By the way, not a single thing sent by the *Gloucester Castle* has arrived yet. I told Mr. Smith to wire direct to Lord Methuen.)

Lady Paget's is a beautifully organised hospital—on a hill about a mile out of Skoplje. They have 350 beds, and could expand in an emergency to 1000. Lady Paget is the 'soul' of the place. I have *lent* them three of our new nurses. It really is a place to be proud of and so beautifully situated with glorious views of the hills. There is a first rate laboratory, and they have their own carpenters' shop and mechanics and everything'. Skoplje itself is very interesting;—quite Turkish. Dr. Maitland took me in yesterday, and it was interesting walking through the bazaars. It is all quite different to Northern Serbia.

P.S.—By the way, I bought that yoke of oxen for Kraguievatz. It was quite necessary.

Valjevo, 15th, August 1915.

I wrote last week from Skoplje, and this is just a little note to say 1 left there on Wednesday night. Dr. Morrison and Dr. Turner, the surgeon he got at Belgrade, arriving on Wednesday morning. Lady Paget telegraphed that Dr. McDougal and her party had arrived at Salonika, and were travelling up in the same train as she. They made a record journey, arriving in Kraguievatz a fortnight from the day they left Southampton.

I wanted very much to come straight here and see if Dr. Hutchison would help, but I thought it better to place the new people first. This I did on Friday morning, and went on to Mladanovatz by car that afternoon, and on here on Saturday.

This is a very fine camp, and the committee may be very proud of it. Sir Ralph writes to me that he inspected Dr. Hutchison's camp, and that he 'has nothing but praise for it.' It really is a splendid piece of organisation.

The staff all looked well, and there is an enormous amount of superfluous energy, as there is in all the British Units here!

I go back by Lazarovatz tomorrow, and see them fairly started. I'll send you a report about that as soon as possible. Then I shall stop at Mladanovatz on my way back, and see how it is working.

This is such a lovely place. I seem to say that in every letter—

wherever I write from! But it is perfectly true, Serbia is a lovely country. We are right up among the hills here; and on this grey and rather misty morning—we might be in Scotland. Could any Scotswoman say anything more? But the blue blue skies and the glorious sunshine are all Serbia.

P.S.—The *Gloucester Castle* things have not arrived yet. Sir Ralph has wired to Lord Methuen about them; and Mr. Behrens in charge of our stores at Salonika will send someone over if we do not hear soon.

Mladanovatz 13th September 1915.

. . . . I have all sorts of interesting things to tell the committee this week.

First about the opening of the fountain here. This took place last Tuesday. Colonel Gentitch and Colonel Michalovitz came up from Kraguievatz for it. We came up in two cars—our seven-seater and an ambulance car belonging to the government. We started at 6 a.m. We *meant* to start at 5 a.m., but that was quite good for this dear, unpunctual country. It is curious how one gets used to things. You remember I told you what an awful road it was, the first time Mrs. Haverfield and I came here with the colonel to choose the site. Positively this time I thought the road quite good! It was a much colder, greyer day than last time, but still very beautiful, and we all enjoyed it. We got here at a quarter to ten, having stopped for coffee at Topola, and Colonel Gentitch went round the camp, which was awfully nice and neat, and then at eleven we went to the fountain.

It was a dedication ceremony, five Greek priests performed it. All the Bevis Camp (the 1st British Field Ambulance Corps), and all our people who could be spared, and Serbian officers representing the artillery, the cavalry, and the infantry, about twenty of them—and some engineer officers, friends of the architects, and the squad of men who did the actual building. The fountain is between the camp and the village, on the same hill, looking right across to Kosmai, the mountain where they fought one of their big battles last year.

A table covered with a white cloth stood in front of the fountain, and on it a silver crucifix, a bowl of water, a long brown candle, lighted, and stuck in a tumbler full of sand, and two bunches of basil, one fresh and one dried. The priests in their

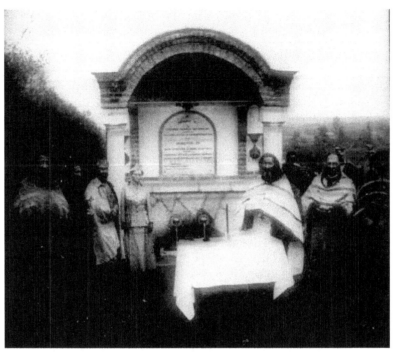

DEDICATION CEREMONY FOR THE FOUNTAIN AT MLADANOVATZ

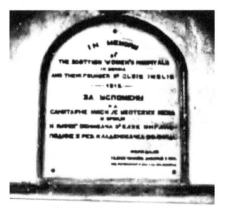

INSCRIPTION
In memory of the Scottish Women's Hospitals in Serbia
And their founder Dr Elsie Inglis–1915

canonicals ranged themselves behind the table, and Colonel R——, who is in command here, and Colonel Gentitch, and Colonel B——, the head of the Medical Department, stood facing them, and all the rest of us, round about. Quite unconsciously we all got together on the right, the Bevis people and us, and the Serbian officers on the left, which was just as well when it came to the blessing and sprinkling with the Holy Water. It would have made an awful muddle if we had all been mixed up. The very first thing that happened was so impressive with them all standing together like that.

The service was intoned, and at the first note, just as if it had been a word of command, each man swept off his cap. and crossed himself—just in a flash, like drill. They cross themselves the opposite way to Catholics, from right to left. The singing of the service was very beautiful; the priests passed the books from one to another, singing alone, and then together. A peasant, dressed in ordinary rough peasant clothes, swung the censer towards us and the others and the priests, and whenever it was swung towards any side the people there bowed. The service went on, and the crucifix was dipped in the bowl for some time. They blessed King Peter of Serbia, Nicholas, Tsar of Russia, and George, King of England.

Then they turned round and blessed the fountain, sprinkling the water on it with the bunch of fresh basil, first in front, and then all round to the back. After that, one of the priests made an address, of which, of course, we understood nothing except Lady Paget's name; but later on Colonel Michalovitz translated it into French, and it was a very pretty little speech, saving how grateful they were to the Scottish Women's Hospitals, and that they are a poor people, and cannot do big things, but they had done this little thing to show they were grateful, and to keep the name of the hospitals 'forever' in the countryside, so that the peasants always would remember. When Lady Paget was ill the peasants prayed in all the country in their little houses for her recovery. Happily I wasn't ill. but they would pray for blessing, all the same. Wasn't it all prettily put?

Colonel Michalovitz stood in the middle and said it all to me, and I felt, as a Suffragist who can speak, I ought to make a speech in reply! But in the first place I should have had to speak in French, and in the second I knew they weren't used to women speaking, so I just said I thanked them a thousand times, and they did not seem to expect anything more.

However, I have run ahead, for Colonel Michalovitz did not make his translation till later. After the fountain had been blessed, and the address given, the priest came to the front of the table, holding the crucifix in his left hand and the basil in his right, and all the officers there went up one by one, beginning with Colonel Gentitch, and the priest sprinkled the water from the basil on their heads, and they kissed the crucifix, and some of them his hand. Then he went round to where the squad of men stood, and sprinkled them, but just walking along in front of them, not individually.

Dr. McGregor had invited the commanding officers, about fifteen of them, to lunch, and we all came back together. Unfortunately there was not room to have the Bevis people too. They had made the mess tent so awfully pretty with red berries, and Charlie—their Austrian cook, who was a waiter at the Trocadero when the war broke out, and had been eighteen months under a chef produced the most *recherché* lunch! Colonel Gentitch proposed my health and the director through Colonel Michalovitz, (for he could speak French), proposed Dr. McGregor's, and altogether the whole thing was most successful. Two of the priests came up to lunch and one of them sang Serbian songs to us afterwards. I do wish you could all have been here. It seems such a shame that we should see all these interesting things and have all the interesting work and you should have all the drudgery at home. *Everybody literally*, here envies us our committee. Your thorough organisation and your abundant supplies and constant helpfulness makes us hear very often, 'If only we had your committee.'

We have got your papers about organisation and shall try to live up to them. They strike me as excellent. And will you tell Mrs. Walker that the Swastika sign on our bales and boxes is blessed by everybody who has to do with equipment, British and Serbian alike. It makes it so easy to pick out our boxes.

The second interesting thing is the work at Lazarovatz. Colonel Gentitch said he would come on there, after the opening of the fountain, however, he found he could not. But Colonel Michalovitz came. Colonel Gentitch and the others went back in the government car, and Dr. McDougal, Colonel Michalovitz and I went on in the seven-seater. Colonel Michalovitz is a splendid man for getting things done, and we spent the whole of the morning going round with him (next morning). As I told you, the hospital at Lazarovatz is housed in various houses in the village, private houses, and inns. I don't know if the censor will let this pass but as I want the red blankets. I *must* tell you the number of beds! We are expected to be ready for 600 beds there. The director has arranged that we shall have charge of the store and the laundry *for the whole hospital*, so we are responsible for the care of the whole equipment.

They are having quite a rush of work, considering how healthy the country is. One day a division passed through and left a hundred sick behind them. This more than filled every bed we had ready. So you can imagine our feelings the next evening when we suddenly heard that fifty more were coming down the line. It was really like war work, *as one imagines it!* We went and turned out a *gast* house, people who had been sitting there in the *café* helping to clear out the tables and chairs, the proprietors helping too, and showing us where extra wood was to be had, and so on. We swept the whole place out to the light of storm lanterns, made a roaring fire, got on some boiling water in the little kitchen place, and then down on us came the patients, beds, bedding, all together. Some of the men were really ill and all of them were dead tired.

Fortunately Serbian beds are made more quickly than our iron ones. Mrs. Haverfield came down in the nick of time with all our house orderlies. We packed that house as no English Hospital would ever dare to pack! But we got a bed for each man. There was no question of bathing, of course! We just tore off their uniforms and their heavy muddy boots. Dr. McDougal wandered round with tea, which they love (they had had their rations all day and weren't hungry, but they gulped down the tea), and it was good to see them sink back on their pillows, saying, '*Leppo, Sestra. Leppo,*' which means, 'It is beautiful. Sister, beautiful.'

Kraguievatz, 26th September 1915.
There are all sorts of exciting things to tell the committee, so I am glad to have the opportunity of sending this home by Sister B———. You probably know more of what is going on at

home than we do here—but the last week has become full of rumours. What seems to be certain is that Bulgaria is mobilising—probably to attack Serbia; that Greece and Roumania are also mobilising—object unknown; and that an Austrian—some say German force is massing on the frontier, and that there is certain to be an attack on Belgrade. I travelled up from Nish yesterday, and the whole line was blocked with trains full of soldiers and transport. We took twenty-one hours on the journey; started at eight o'clock at night and got here at five o'clock the next afternoon—dead tired!

Last week Austrian aeroplanes were 'announced,' and the authorities evidently believed the report; for the Arsenal was emptied of workmen—and they don't stop work willingly just now. So—as a Serbian officer said to me yesterday—'Serbia is exactly where she was a year ago.' It does seem hard lines on our little Ally. If only they could have sent a British Expeditionary Force up here this summer, it would have made absolutely all the difference—all the Balkan States would have declared on our side, Germany could not have got ammunition through to the Turks, and probably things would have been easier for Russia. I suppose one ought not to criticise—but to lengthen our line in France and have muddling diplomacy out here! Of course I believe we have poured in money and munitions and stores—but an Army Corps would have simply solved the situation.

Well, as to how this affects us. Sir Ralph was talking about the various possibilities. As long as the Serbians fight we'll stick to them—retreat if necessary, burning all our stores. If they are overwhelmed we must escape—probably *via* Montenegro. Don't worry about us. We won't do anything rash or foolish; and it you will trust us to decide, as we must know most about the situation out here, will act rationally.

Colonel Harrison was dining here last night and says there are developments in the political situation, and we must all be ready for work immediately. We are awfully worried at the *Gloucester Castle* equipment not arriving for if there is any rush I am afraid we shall be short of dressing's.

Colonel Gentitch is coming up with me next week to see Mladanovatz, Lazarovatz, and Valjevo. Your telegram has come about calling Mladanovatz 'The Neil Fraser Hospital.' and you will see from the enclosed letter that he is very pleased. He spoke about

177

it the other night too.

Mr. Smith is going over to Malta to try and find that lost equipment.....

We have succeeded in getting the cesspool closed altogether, and are using the bucket system. Huz and Buz—the two oxen we bought—do the carting. Such a funny thing, we had to sign a special Act to have them called Huz and Buz! It seemed their Serbian names were something else, and you cannot alter an ox's name without an Act. I laughed till I cried, and now an orderly comes up, to salute and say solemnly something about the fodder for 'Hooz and Booz.' I believe Dr. Chesney has carefully explained to the whole hospital that they are Biblical characters, but what they make of it all I don't know. When we had bought our own they sent us down two more from the Military Hospital, which is *so* like them, and they were promptly named Gog and Magog; but I have said those; must be strictly pet names, for I am not going to sign Acts for altering the names of government oxen.

Mladanovatz, 29th Sept. 1915.

Mr. Smith is still in Malta hunting for the *Gloucester Castle* things. I my hear of them when I go in to Kraguievatz this afternoon. I must go to see Colonel Gentitch about things for Lazarovatz, wood for a new laundry, etc., and also the winter plans for here—but I shall come up again tomorrow for the operations.

...I meant to stay at Nish only one day, but it took so long to get all the things collected at the Red Cross Store that I had to stay two. Sir Ralph has established the most delightful Rest House at Nish for the use of the units, just opposite the station, in little white temporary buildings. It is such a comfort—the cleanliness and orderliness. An American turned up one afternoon while I was there, and sank into a deckchair, exclaiming, 'How neat and English!' It is a most interesting place to stay in—all sorts and conditions of Britishers drop in and out, going one way and another. I saved up some nice things I heard for the committee.

Of these let us give one: A man from another unit working in Serbia, during a conversation with Dr. Inglis poured out his woes with regard to the dissensions in his unit. He wound up by saying, "I sup-

pose you never have these troubles—you seem such a happy family!"
Dr. Inglis writes:

I looked at him, to see if he was laughing. But he wasn't. He
was in dead earnest. So I hid my smile and said, 'Well, perhaps
women can manage other women better than men can!'

And so "the long, peaceful summer" drew to a close. In the last letters we can hear the brewing of the storm that was so soon to develop
Serbia.

Valjevo

Dr. Hutchison's letters which follow carry us back again to the
month of April, when she with her unit, closely following on
Dr. Inglis' departure, sailed for Serbia from Cardiff. They tell the
story of this particular unit from the day of its starting until it
left Valjevo.

S.S. Ceramic, off Coast of Spain,
Friday.

After the last handkerchief-wavings at the Caledonian Station
things went wonderfully smoothly, up to our arriving at Cardiff.

That night we spent in the docks, and only finally set sail next
morning at 9.30. What a strange and unforgettable send off we
had, one which will live in the memory for all time. To me it
was so strongly suggestive of the influence of the war drawing
us all nearer to our fellow creatures, known and unknown.

Well, to describe our send-off, having first piqued your curiosity about it.

We first caught sight of some army nursing sisters, who, we
soon learnt, had been prompted by a kindly feeling to give us
a heartening send-off. As we moved slowly into the dock, I realised that quite a crowd was gathering, and not a known face
among them. Dock labourers seemed to rise out of the ground
so quickly did their numbers swell. Grimy and untidy in their
working garb, they still were to me a more welcome sight than
any well-dressed crowd. Next came 'Tommies,' strolling along
from odd corners till quite a company of them had assembled.
A number of these seated themselves on a suspended chain and
regaled us with 'Tipperary' and other songs—Welsh, Scotch,
and English, we in turn fully contributed our share. Jests were

shouted up from the shore and quickly replied to by the more nimble tongues among us.

From the shore came: 'Are we down-hearted?' To which we replied with suitable vigour: 'No! No!! No!!!' 'Are we going to win?' shouted the crowd on the shore. 'Yes!' we frantically cried. So the time quickly passed as the water rose in the dock, till a most unexpected anticlimax came with the snapping of the chain and also the precipitation of a struggling mass of 'Tommies' on the ground. To this we shouted from our Olympic heights, 'Encore!' And still the waters rose, and an increasing inclination showed itself among the 'Tommies' to cast off light music and jests and to blend their voices more and more insistently in a plaintive 'Song of Farewell.'

Intervals came, when ringing cheers were raised for us, to which the chief medical officer replied by voicing the thanks of the company: but the 'Song of Farewell' became more and more the dominant note. At last the gates were opened and the *Ceramic* took her stately course towards the open sea and the unknown. A few last cheers were raised, but were quickly subdued by the 'Song of Farewell,' which floated over the waters to us till it became only a faint wail in the far distance.

. . . . We are all a very harmonious company, and each person seems bent on making the expedition a big success.

Camerata, Sirada, Mercani,
Malta, 8th May.

I seldom set out to do one thing, without tackling something quite unexpected on the way, therefore instead of now being somewhere near Salonika *en route* for Serbia, I am working with my unit in a British Military Hospital at Malta. At this moment I am sitting in the entrance courtyard of our hospital, waiting for the arrival of a fresh contingent of wounded. We have the good fortune to be working in the building which was in the fifteenth century the hospital of the Knights of St. John. Now it is merely called the Valetta Military Hospital, but those who have the inner eye open, realise the immense attraction of working in a building of such historic interest. Entering by the rather insignificant doorway, you find yourself in a large, square, flagged courtyard.

Brightly coloured flowers grow in what may have formerly

been the central fountain, and clamber up the walls to touch the balustraded balcony. By the arched entrance at the far end you go down a flight of stairs and then proceed along wide whitewashed corridors till you enter the gigantic wards one of which holds 90 patients comfortably. So thick are the immense walls that on the hottest day the air is deliciously cool in every part of the building. Quaint little recesses indicate that the building is not modern, and the heavily barred windows of the slaves' dungeons tell their own tale; but indeed the whole atmosphere is charged with scents of the olden days. Where formerly the Knights of St. John in their flowing white robes, tended their sick folk, may now be seen, moving among the beds, four painfully modern women doctors in their painfully modern ward coats! Alas! why *are* we so keen for the times to move on.

You will, however, want a few words of explanation on the situation. Well, we had been here three days when we were summoned into the governor's presence (after a preliminary interview with the P.M.O.) and it was explained to us that the services of the unit were very urgently required, as a sudden and unforeseen strain was going to be put on the medical organisation

We liked our chief from the first moment we set eyes on him, and we think he should get a D.S.O for the splendid way he has organised the hospital at short notice. Guess who our patients are? The men who have been wounded at the Dardanelles—a mixture of Australians and Britishers. It is lovely to have the chance of looking after our own men for a bit, and I have been thrilled and appalled at the accounts they give us of the landing of our troops on the peninsula of Gallipoli; but I expect us wiser not to write about it. The Australians arrived here first and are very interesting as a character study, though it's early days to sum them up. When the second batch came, I said to one man, 'Are you Australian too?' The reply was, 'No, just plain British.'

15th. We are all saddened because of a death we had today. He was an Australian, and a more friendly, plucky young fellow I have never seen. He had repeated haemorrhage from a wound in his arm, which had finally to he amputated yesterday. He was game to the last, and all the convalescents stood to attention when an hour or two later he was carried from the ward covered with the Union Jack. It doesn't sound much, but I'll never forget it. Nor shall I forget another man, whom I also found in the early hours, pulseless but conscious. Literally with his dying breath he reassured me: 'Honestly, you know, doctor, I'm perfectly fit.'

One glories in such pluck, and yet one loathes war more and more every day, because it makes you see everything through blood and tears. I won't write more today. We sail for Serbia on Saturday next, and it will cost us a big pang to say goodbye to our British Tommies. I'm so glad, *ever* so glad, to have had this little chance of serving them and mothering them, and it's a great joy to us that they should so quickly be enthusiastic about their women doctors.

The Australians and New Zealanders we found delightfully frank and easy to get on with. They were always ready to jeer at the sentimental effusion of the *Malta Chronicle* over 'our wounded heroes.' When an Australian was asked one day where he had managed to get a coat he was sporting, the quick reply came: 'Pinched it from another wounded hero, doctor!'

Dr. Hutchison and her unit remained in Malta until they were wired for from Serbia, where they were urgently needed.

That they did good work in Malta is shown the letter of appreciation written by the governor, Lord Methuen, after the unit's departure:

> San Antonio Palace, Malta.
> Dear Sir.—As I have written to Sir Ralph Paget, it is not in my power to express my gratitude sufficiently for the help given me by the Serbian Unit. There came the first avalanche of wounded, and no further aid from home was due for a fortnight, so, sooner than see my men neglected in order to nurse Serbians, I took it on myself to detain the unit for one night. They leave here blessed by myself, surgeons, nurses and patients alike, for they have proved themselves most capable and untiring workers. They never made the smallest difficulty, and would not have been sorry had I ordered them to remain another week.—Yours truly,
> 23/5/15.   (Sgd.)   Methuen. G.M.

What an eventful day! This is the day on which our first tent has been pitched. I am now sitting in it, so as to be at hand and superintend everything. Our camp is on the slope of the hill just above the hospital where we are at present living. It has a glorious look towards the immense semicircle of hills in the shelter of which Valjevo lies. In the heat haze of mid-day I can only guess the outline of the distant high, hills, but in sunset lights they stand out so proudly in their serene blue, a joy to the eye and food for the soul. I shall describe the camp to you when it is all pitched and ready for work. I am longing to see the lines of white tents, and the flags waving, and patients tucked into nice clean beds with pretty red coverlets. At 7 a.m. this morning five of us were here to watch the first tent go up under the skilful manipulation of our 'handy men'

We had no bottle of champagne and no speech to mark the portentous moment. We only stood around in apparent curiosity, but it seemed to me there was a touch of awe and reverence in the atmosphere as, with a flap of her wings, our first tent rose to her full height an emblem of hope and wonder. As a white-sailed ship sets forth eagerly for strange ports, so it seemed to me our first solitary tent symbolised the position of our unit. Into what unknown regions was it going, for how long, and to what end? Time only could answer these questions, so we turned our attention to the business in hand.

I somehow feel that our adventure is going to work out happily, and I shall write soon to tell you all about the camp.

Valjevo, 15th June 1915.

. . . We are now hurrying forward our camp, and Campfield and McAllan are working their hardest with a lot of Austrian prisoners. The position as regards work is as follows: Typhus is getting steadily less, and all the cases are being dealt with in one hospital (the one in which we are staying as guests). It is almost certain that we shall not have typhus to deal with at present, but get medical cases first, and surgical work whenever the advance takes place. I find we have really been sent here to be ready for the Serbian advance, which is expected to take place at any time. It is fully expected that there will be a recrudescence of

---

1. Dr. Hutchison's letters continued.

typhus in winter, so if we are still here then we shall have to deal with it. . . .

Miss Jack is a splendid administrator, and I do think the unit should run with the minimum of friction. We have started a camp journal and a bugle, and I intend to organise fortnightly entertainments whenever the work allows of it. It's a great thing to keep people happy, and I should like the thing to be a success.

Valjevo, July 1915.

. . . . . Our wards look very well indeed, and are fortunately the coolest of all the tents, as they are so large and we can take the sides entirely away and allow whatever breeze there is to blow through. The smaller tents get unpleasantly hot during the day-time but we have fortunately got some *ladnaks*, where we repair when not otherwise occupied. *Ladnaks* are of various sizes, but they are all built on the same principle. A supply of wood in the shape of young tress and cut branches is brought in, and the trunks are stuck into deeply cut holes in the ground to form any size or shape of shelter. Other trunks are then placed from post to post lengthways and crossways, and firmly nailed to form a roof, and on the roof are piled the cut branches.

The result is a delightfully cool retreat on hot days, in any part where trees are lacking. I must give you a little description of our camp. Valjevo itself nestles in a long dip between two hills, while we are on the lower slopes of one of them. Leaving the town of Valjevo, one follows a broad road which slants upwards to a plateau, on which stands the 3rd Reserve Hospital, which gave us food and shelter for close on three weeks. The plateau in its turn soon slopes upward, and from the hospital gate one sees an imposing array of tents up the hillside and flags flutter-ing from two tall poles in the foreground, A generous extent of ground has been ringed in with barbed wire, and visitors are challenged at the entrance gate by the sentry before being allowed to proceed up the newly made road to the encamp-ment.

The road ends at the C.M.O.'s office tent, from which stretch, on the right hand side, the remainder of the office and other working tents; on the left stands the big mess tent, with a large *ladnak* in front of it; and farther up the hill the cook-house, storeroom, and sleeping quarters. Beyond this collection of tents comes a clear space, then down the farther slope are the six big ward marquees, and still farther down the slope, wash-house, patients' kitchen, receiving and bath tents, and the arrangements for the destruction of refuse.

At the back of our tents is a fairly large orchard, which has been rented for us, and where members repair freely in off-duty time, for the heat is really very intense.

I shall be able to tell you more about the work and the patients in my next letter. So far my colleagues have done the medical work, and I have only come in touch with a few serious cases apart from my usual round of inspection. My day is spent in flying about from one side of the camp to the other, with an occasional walk down to the 3rd Reserve Hospital to enlist the help of the director, who has been told off to assist me in every possible way.

One morning before 7 a.m., when the whole camp was astir with the energy of a beehive after having enjoyed its first night under canvas and was anticipating the pleasure of its first camp breakfast, an enormous bird (a French biplane) came into sight and began to wheel and curve above our heads, then finally settled on the plateau below us. The C.M.O. tried to continue a business conversation with the carpenter, till the carpenter began to move downhill, and finally with a most expressive, 'Oh, *Gospodgitza!*' ('Oh, Madam!'), broke into a run, followed by the C.M.O., the cook with a kitchen ladle in her hand, the sanitary inspector with her broom, and all the other members of the unit. John Gilpin's flight was mild compared to ours. . . .

Nothing gives me so strongly a sense of topsy-turvydom in the universe as the presence of Austrian orderlies in our camp both for hospital and house service. To become familiar with the blue uniform under such novel circumstances gives me a feeling of the creeps sometimes. To have it in one's tent, scrubbing the floor, filling and emptying one's bath, and doing many kindly offices, to see it in the wards giving kindly care and attention to its own enemy—these are sights which I never quite get used to. It keeps me in constant remembrance of our own men in a similar capacity; one wonders whether perhaps they too may not have just such offices to perform, and so one does all one can to make life as pleasant as one can for them.

One of the prettiest touches in our camp life is the friendship which has sprung up between McAllan, our handy man, and one of the prisoners, a young Hungarian boy called Michael. Michael calls McAllan '*Vater*,' and though he speaks an (to me at least) incomprehensible muddle of German, and McAllan speaks broad Scotch, they have no difficulty in understanding one another. One often sees them sitting side by side on a packing-case after working hours having a heart-to-heart talk. One night, as they were separating, McAllan was overheard to say, 'well a've enjoyed your crack fine, Michael, but a just wisht a'd kent what ye was talkin' aboot.' Delicious, isn't it?

McAllan is really a treat, and has become absolutely indispensable to me. His favourite axiom is that broad Scotch is the best means of making oneself understood in Serbia! ...

August 1915.

As I went today to pay my morning visit to the invalids in the orchard, different companies of soldiers dashed into the orchard from various points and then dropped on one knee with raised rifles, prepared to fire at an unseen foe. Then one realised sharply once again that, in spite of all the joy of autumnal days, the fight one had just seen in our peaceful orchard was being played in earnest over almost the whole of the civilised world. . . . There is no longer the silence and restraint of the early days. A lively chatter is ample testimony that the men no longer feel themselves to be in foreign surroundings, but are very much at home with the various *Sestrae*, and looking forward to being soon *kod kuche*.

Those two words mean 'at home,' and are interwoven with the days of work in Serbia. One day a patient was clamouring loudly to be allowed to go *kod kuche*, when I heard a voice murmur at my side, '*Kod kuche*.' Looking round, I found the speaker was an Austrian orderly who was evidently (from the look in his eyes) seeing beyond patients and hospital wards to his own little home in a quiet Austrian valley. Perhaps others, the patients and Austrian orderlies sometimes murmur '*Kod kuche*,' and see invisible things.

When night falls the red-swathed lumps glow in the darkness, throwing a strange glamour over the sleeping patients and the watching figures of sisters and orderlies. Then one sees the invisible, as one recalls the long ward with its crimson-shaded electric lights at Valetta Hospital, and one's thoughts stretch out to feel the touch of the international. Surely it is hardly possible for Britisher and Serb to arrive at a mutual kindly understanding with laugh and gesture and isolated words (appropriate or inappropriate), and then part to be as if they had never met. One likes rather to think that when we leave the hillside once again silent, with brown, grassless areas alone speaking of its former more bustling existence, that we shall have left more lasting imprints in the shape of a wider international understanding sympathy.

The enteric tents have been to me the most interesting. It has been a great joy to see many serious cases come round the corner, don the blue convalescent suits, and then join the happy throng going *kod kuche*. The blue convalescents suits are greatly coveted by the patients, and each man bequeaths his to a pal before he leaves. The suits are, in fact, booked a week or two in advance. One gets some quaint votes of thanks, and one man wrote a poem to Dr. Philips, the refrain being in the of 'Mother, my Mother.'

September 1915

The camp has been inspected by several people—among them the Head of the Serbian Sanitary Department and the Head of all the French Missions in Serbia. The most recent visitors were Sir Ralph and Lady Paget, who expressed themselves as more than satisfied with everything. During their stay I had the interesting experience of dining with them first at a medical dinner and then at an army dinner. The army dinner was quite a big thing—very prettily arranged in a large hall. I had there the honour of conversing with the big Serbian field-marshal whose name will be handed to posterity as the saviour of Serbia from the Austrians. He asked whether he might do himself the honour of visiting the camp, to which I of course replied that the honour would be mine!

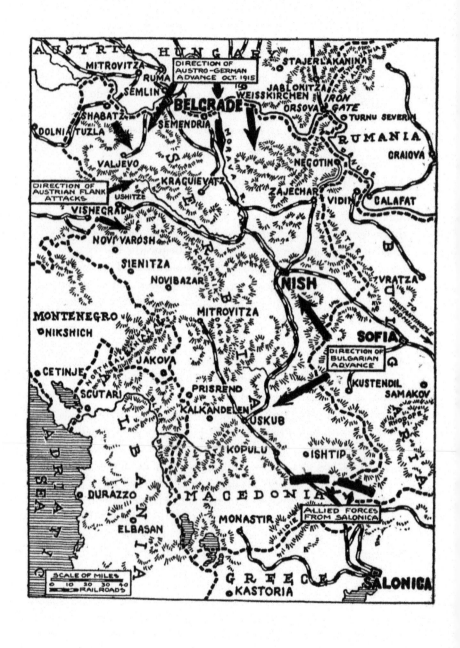

CHAPTER 4

The Great Retreat

The "long-drawn-out fight with typhus" had ended in April—
"the peaceful summer" was drawing to a close—when in November
the storm of the German-Austrian invasion burst over Serbia. The line
of hospitals in the north at Mladanovatz, Lazarovatz, and Valjevo was
ordered hastily to retreat. Mladanovatz and Lazarovatz evacuated in
an incredibly short time packed their equipment and came down to
Kraguievatz, where Dr. Inglis was. From there the Lazarovatz women
with Dr. Inglis' party had to make a further evacuation to Krushevatz, this time losing most of their equipment. Dr. McGregor and her
party were taken from Kraguievatz to Kralievo, from which place they
joined the Great Retreat. Dr. Hutchison's Unit in the meantime were
first taken to Pojega, and then moved to Vrinjatcha Banja. On Sir
Ralph Paget's recommendation the women were given the choice of
going home if they desired with the parties who were attempting a
trek across the Albanian Mountains, or staying behind at their posts.
Both Dr. Inglis and Dr. Hutchison decided to stay, and with them a
number of their staff. These were all taken prisoners by the enemy
in the month of November. The rest, who desired to go home were
formed into two parties under Mr. Smith and Dr. McGregor, and successfully accomplished the Great Retreat.

LETTER FROM DR. INGLIS, BROUGHT BY MR. SMITH

Kraguievatz, 5th November 1915,
. . . . Just in case Mr. Smith gets home, this is a little line to the
committee to explain where we are, and what is happening.
We in the very centre of the storm, and it is anything, but pleasant to be part of a beaten and retreating army. All our hospitals,

189

planned as part of a campaign on the Danube, have had to be evacuated. The first to be moved was Dr. McGregor's, immediately after the fall of Belgrade. This was inevitable, lying as Mladanovatz does on the line from there. She and Miss Pares performed really a feat—packed in two days and got the *whole* of their equipment down. They were stationed Kraguievatz, in the Artillery Barracks, to open a hospital for slightly wounded and a huge dressing-station.

They organised magnificently, and had 600 beds running, and I think 5000 cases a week through their hands in the fortnight they were working. Then Kraguievatz had to be evacuated. The next to be moved was Dr. Hutchison's. They had more warning, but also got all their goods off. They were sent to, Pojega. But within a week it had to be evacuated the Austrians pouring over the western frontier. That was a surprise (for good soldiers thought that at any rate, this Western Morava valley could be held—especially the western end, with its hills). Dr Hutchison is now at Vrinjatcha Banja, farther east, along the same line, where she has a small hospital and a dressing-station. The Hopes are with her.

Of all our three hospitals in the north, Lazarovatz was the last to be moved—rather puzzling, as it was between the other two; but they expected to be able to hold that bit of ground, evacuating Valjevo without fighting, to shorten the enormously long line they have to defend. In the end, Lazarovatz had also to go, the people leaving in an awful hurry and in awful discomfort. Some day we'll tell you all about it. They were sent here to Krushevatz, have got two big store-houses, and have done good work for the last week, with innumerable dressings.

At Kraguievatz, our hospital filled to the doors, 175 beds instead of the 125 we ought to have, and we took over two '*gast* houses' for convalescents—60 patients more. The sisters worked splendidly, and Mr. Davidson and Dr. McDougal are a capital pair of assistants. (Dr. Chesney was off with the Field Ambulance.) We had 75 new cases to start off with, and from 30 to 40 a day after that, clearing out as quickly as we could—dressing all the morning, operations all the afternoon, and the patients x-rayed on their way to the operating-room. It was heart-breaking work leaving the hospital. We cleared the '*gast* houses,' and sent off every man who could walk, but even so there were left 20 bad cases, with six ignorant orderlies to look after them, and three doctors for all the hospitals together.

We left in two parties, and I went back the last thing to give the men some cigarettes. Already the whole place was in chaos, windows shut, and one man with a long splint, with his splint off, sitting up winding up his bandages. One man with secondary haemorrhage nearly died, and, as everything was packed, I had to have him removed to the Military Hospital with a tourniquet on.

All this will make you understand how I came to the conclusion that if we are really to help the Serbs now, we must stick to our posts. Sir Ralph did not at first agree, and especially felt that we ought to move in order to save our expensive equipment. But when he came to think of it, he realised that in this headlong retreat we cannot save it. We each got our equipment off in the first instance—complete—but it is absolutely impossible to move it now. Sir Ralph, himself, has lost the whole of his, in Nish. Further, the constant feeling that the Foreign hospitals must be saved was only an added worry to the Serbs. Instead of helping, we were adding to the difficulties, and if the committee could have seen Colonel Gentitch's face when I said to him that we were not going to move again, but that they could count on us just where we stood, I think they would have been touched.

Sir Ralph decided that everybody who wanted should go down to Novi-bazar and over into Montenegro, if possible. A party of twenty left here today—five of Dr. Hutchison's, nine of Dr. Hollway's, four Field Ambulance, and two of mine—Mr. Smith goes with them. My matron has since decided to go too!

Dr. McGregor has trekked with her whole party from Kralievo (where she was sent from Kraguievatz to form another dressing-station), and I think intends to form a hospital at Novi-bazar. But we have missed one another every time, and I only know what Miss Pares told me. Getting no answers to our telegrams, and hearing nothing, and with there being no trains, I went up today to Kralievo in the Welsh Ambulance (which is now the Field Ambulance really), to the undisguised distress of the officers at Headquarters! Campfield drove, and we did not see the shadow of a German. Colonel Antitch is left there with 700 wounded—three assistants and no nurses. The dressing-station

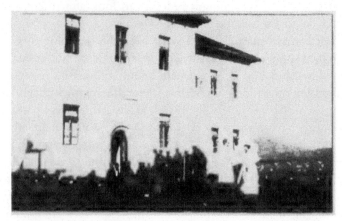

HOSPITAL AT KRALIEVO

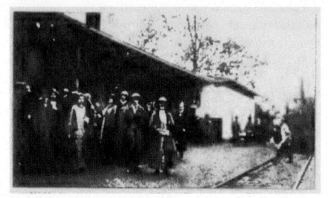

S.W.H. PARTY WAITING THE LAST TRAIN FROM KRALIEVO

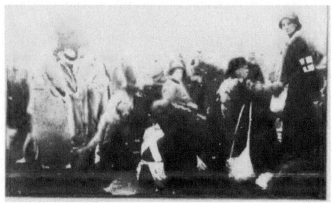

RESTING DURING THE RETREAT

moved two days ago to Rashka—he understood for Novi-bazar, to form a hospital. They have not a scrap of equipment, and cannot get it. Still, the place may be a perfectly good one, and it may be possible to give valuable help in a Serbian hospital.

My 'line' has lengthened. Some day we'll have lots to tell you. Just now one can think of nothing but these poor little people in this awful hole—with the country they have fought so hard for overrun from end to end. They can hardly speak to one without breaking down—even strong men among them. 'They look at one so eagerly, and say, 'When will your men be up?' *When?* The road to Kralievo today was crowded with refugees in their shaky bullock-carts full of all their household things. And there were groups of stragglers from the army. As we came back these men were being gathered up by officers. The whole of Serbia has been thrown back on this Western Morava valley, and now there is nothing left but a further retreat south, and then—surrender? They have lost their heads. There is no denying it. They admit it themselves. And no wonder. It is as bad as Belgium.

I have forgotten to tell you that we have a Hospital here in the gymnasium—200 beds—very nice building, and all our equipment. And we have had charge of an English sailor—Danials—ever since the bombardment of Belgrade, where he was wounded. He is going with Mr. Smith tomorrow.

It is with a feeling of sadness we read of the breaking up of the beautiful camps at Valjevo and Mladanovatz, and the evacuation of the hospital at Lazarovatz—the hospitals into which so much thought and labour and enthusiasm had been put; but we know they had done good work, and were prepared for any amount more. The members of the units who trekked through the mountains gave proof of the enduring powers of women, and those who stayed behind and faced the storm and lived through it were, as Dr. Inglis expressed it, "the fortunate ones." for to them was given the privilege of standing by the Serbian men in their hour of crucifixion—the men of whom it was said by an American Red Cross doctor to the war correspondent of the *Daily Mail* (23rd February 1915):

My word, Clarke, but I tell you these men are great. I feel so small beside them that I could hide myself. Pain! Suffering! You've not seen bravery until you've seen these men suffer. I'd take off a hand, an arm, or a leg—without anaesthetics, mind you, and will the fellow budge?—no, not an eyelid. And if you hear them say '*Kukn lebe*' (Oh dear') that's as much as you hear, and not often that much. And die! They'll die without a sound—unless it is to thank you, if they can, before they go. Where this race of soldiers sprang from I don't pretend to know, but I tell you right now they are God's own men.

Mr. Smith tells the story of the Retreat as it affected some of the S.W.H. women:

For some time rumour had been busy about another invasion, this time by a combined German-Austrian Army, which was known to be massing on the Danube. Ferdinand of Bulgaria, after playing with the Allies till he was ready, at last, to show his hand, declared war on Serbia immediately after the attack of the Austrian-German Army opened on the Danube. Serbia might have held out for a time in the north, but, to meet the new enemy on the Bulgarian frontier, her army, something like 250,000, had to be divided, each section having to face a fresh army of 300,000 strong. Help had been expected from Britain and France, also from Greece. Greece and Serbia were bound by treaty, arranged after the second Balkan War, to help each other in case of invasion by Bulgaria. We all know how Greece kept her promise. So, when her hour of bitter trial came, Serbia stood alone.

News reached us in Kraguievatz in October that Belgrade had fallen, and that the Serbian Army was being hard pressed. We were warned to have all our stores in readiness, as it might be necessary to evacuate the town in a week or ten days. But within twenty-four hours of this warning we got orders to leave Kraguievatz at once, for a town farther south. The situation was now desperate, and the Serbian Army was everywhere in retreat. During all our stay Kraguievatz had been the seat of the Serbian Army Staff, which was now preparing to leave for safer quarters. With the departure of the army chiefs, despair seemed to seize upon the poor people, and there was a wild scramble to escape from the doomed city. Confusion and disorder reigned everywhere.

At no time does the Slav shine as an organiser, but in the time of trouble his talent for disorganisation becomes absolute gen-

194

ius. The sound of the guns had been an everyday experience for us, but they were getting nearer, and the railway was threatened, and no time was to be lost if we were to get clear. We got away with our stores by the last train which left the city, passing through the junction only an hour before it was shelled. We had been ordered to Krushevatz, which had been considered safe, but on arrival we found that it was safe no longer.

After consultation with the Army Authorities it was decided that all foreign missions that wished to get away should make for the Adriatic by Montenegro and Albania, and go south by Monastir to Salonika. The great difficulty was to get the transport. The trains had stopped running, so bullock-wagons were our only hope. We were promised eight. We loaded up six of our wagons, and most of our party got away, that afternoon. My own detachment was to follow the next morning with the remaining two wagons. More delays the next morning! The enemy was now quite close, and shells were falling near the town, which was also being bombed from the air, and the enemy was reported to be but a few miles off.

We finally got away from the hospital about noon, joined the main road, and became part of what was to be known as the Great Retreat. The road was a moving mass of transport of all kinds—motor-wagons, bullock-wagons, horse-wagons, men, and guns, besides the civilian population, men, women, and children, all intent on escape. The country here is undulating-, and the procession, as it dipped into a hollow and reappeared on the crest, to dip and reappear again and again, until it was finally lost as it passed over the distant hills, looked like a great dragon wandering over the countryside. This procession had been passing continuously for days, stretching from one end of Serbia to the other, and one realised that this was something more than an army in retreat: it was the passing of a whole nation into exile, a people leaving a lost country.

It has been said that in all history there is no parallel to this exodus, unless it may be the flight of the Israelites out of the land of Egypt; but in their case the exodus led to freedom—in this, it was a nation going into exile.

We kept going during the daylight, but towards sunset the wagons commenced to draw into the fields by the roadside for a few

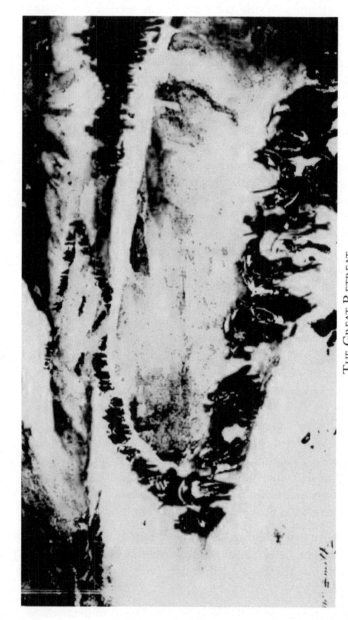

THE GREAT RETREAT

hours' rest. About ten o'clock we took the road again, and as I was anxious to overtake the party which had left the day before, I decided to keep going all night. Rain fell about midnight, and in an hour or two the roads were as only Serbian roads can be. The going became ghastly, the wagons were frequently up to their axles in mud, and breaking down everywhere and causing endless delays. The night was as black as the pit, and the rain got worse, but there was nothing for it but to keep plunging on, sometimes up to the knees in mud and water. In the dark the road was difficult to follow, and wagons fell foul of each other, and got jammed. Here and there someone in authority would come along with a lantern, and try to clear up the confusion. Officers shouted orders, drivers swore at their bullocks, and at each other, tempers gave out, and quarrels were frequent. Weeping women were seen staggering along with babies in their arms or carrying the pitiful remains of their household goods. Everyone was soaked to the skin, and sick at heart, but there was nothing for it but to stumble on, praying for the dawn.

Dawn came at last, and with it the promise of a better day, and an hour or two afterwards we came upon our party, which had started twenty-four hours ahead of us, and who were preparing breakfast. A good meal and all our troubles of the night before assumed their proper perspective. The sun was shining when we took the road again, and there seemed something in living after all. We kept going all day, and about eight in the evening pitched our camp in the outskirts of a village, glad to lie down after a march—bar three hours' rest of the night before—of thirty-six hours.

We took seven days to reach Prishtina, sleeping mostly in the open, if the weather was not too bad. One wet night we got shelter in the house of a mountain *gendarme*—a bleak outpost on a hilltop, which might at a pinch have held a dozen with comfort, but over thirty weary souls thought themselves lucky to get inside. At Prishtina we hoped to get instructions about the route we were to take, but nothing definite could be fixed. Rumour was busy that day in the town about the advance of the Allied Army—the French and British Force—which, as a matter of fact, was itself at that moment in retreat towards Salonika. Next morning we left for Prisrem, where the Army Headquarters Staff had gone, and where definite orders about our route would be issued.

That days march led us over the fated Plain of Kosovo, where centuries ago the old Serbs, under the great Czar Lazar, the hero of a hundred ballads, made their last stand and fell before the onrush of the Turk. Serbia was now staggering under the heaviest blow since this great battle five hundred years before. At Prisrem we found many members of different multi-nations, French, Russian, and British, who like ourselves, were finding a way to the coast. The route *via* Albania and Monastir to Salonika was pronounced impossible, as the one available road was now in the hands of the Bulgars, so our only way led over the snow clad mountains of Montenegro and the Albanian Alps. The Serbian Headquarters Staff was here, and many of the Foreign Diplomats, amongst them the French Minister, all trying to get clear. So this route was our only hope, and we set about getting what provisions we could.

By this time food was unpleasantly scarce, and famine prices were the rule. Everybody was searching for food, and one day I met two British officers whom I knew——one an admiral, carrying a big tin of biscuits, and a colonel with a tin of bully beef under either arm. Both hailed me cheerfully and displayed their good luck.

Everything was now ready, so we set out for Ipek, where we were to leave our bullock-wagons, buy ponies, to cross the mountains of Montenegro and Albania to the Adriatic. The day began badly for us. From the start we were in difficulties with our oxen, and we found out later that the poor beasts had got little or nothing to eat at Prisrem, and were now starving. The rest of the procession was soon far ahead of us. I managed to buy some hay at a roadside farm, but our beasts were too weak to go far, and in the end we had to give them to an Albanian at a wayside farmhouse. By this time it was dark and we were miles behind the rest of our party, so there was no hope for it but to keep going all night.

After one wagon was drawn up a hill, we had to unhitch the oxen and go back with them to help up their weaker brethren. This went on the whole night long and hills were all too frequent, and it was a tired and sorry-looking party which crawled into a small town, the name of which I cannot remember. We rested here for a day, partly for the sake of the beasts, partly for our own, and set out again next morning, hoping to get to Ipek the following day. That night we rested in the Monastery of Dechani. This monastery, one of the biggest in the world, was full of refugees making, like ourselves, for Ipek. Through the kindness of one of the priests we got tea on arrival, and a room to ourselves, which the priest told us we might find rather cold, but all the rest of the bedding was lost. It was savagely cold, and we shut the windows, to find next morning that we were in a newly built part of the monastery, and the windows had as yet, no glass in them.

Towards the end of the thirtieth day we reached Ipek, and obtained quarters in a Military Barracks. The great difficulty now was to get horses, as the government had been commandeering all available beasts for transport purposes. The refugees were glad to get beasts at any price, and the Albanian horse-dealers of Ipek had been having the time of their lives and reaping a rare harvest. It took me the better part of three days to get the number we required. After buying fifteen ponies we set about getting provisions, for no food of any kind could be bought while crossing the mountains. Snow was falling when we turned out the next morning, and looked likely to continue. This was the first big snowstorm of the year, and we had been in hopes of crossing the mountains before it came. The ponies were loaded up, and we got away from Ipek about ten. We knew we were in for a long day's march, as no camping was possible, except at one place far ahead.

We had now tackled the most trying part of our march, and should the snow continue, it would mean disaster and death to thousands. As we went on, the track became narrower, with just enough room for the pony with pack to pass along. The snow continued for hours. The going was fairly good at first, but later on in the day, as it grew colder, our difficulties increased. There were thousands of refugees and ponies ahead of us, and with all this traffic the paths became hard and icy. The track was at one time at the bottom of the pass, alongside the rushing river, then there would be a sharp rise, and it would wind its way in and out to the top of the pass, with the rushing river now far below. By this time the going was more than difficult, and the greatest care was necessary, especially downhill.

One horse fell over, and literally rolled into the river, luckily at a place not far above the stream, and after some trouble it was got out, looking little the worse. Others were not so fortunate, and the day's march cost the life of many a poor beast which fell into a place where it was impossible to lend help. Sometimes a merciful bullet would put an end to its suffering, but as often as not it was left to die where it fell. Progress was slow. At awkward corners the ponies had to be slowly led one by one, and this meant await of an hour or more in the bitter cold till one's turn came, often at a place where it was impossible to go forward or turn back.

Night came down when we were far from our camping-ground, and a great part of this trying march was done in the dark. Ticklish work leading a pony on a dark night down a narrow icy path, with a high cliff on one side, and nothing but a dark abyss on the other, with a rushing river far below; but the mountain pony is very surefooted, and it is better to leave him to take his own way. During this part of the Retreat the plight of the Austrian prisoners, captured in the battle of a year ago, was terrible. They were shepherded in great bands before the retreating Serbian Army.

At last we reached our camping-ground. A few of our party had already arrived, though the majority were still struggling through the pass, but to our great relief all arrived safely, and we set about preparing supper. Trees had been felled and fires were burning everywhere, and the scene amidst the snow was unforgettable. A party of peasants invited us to their roaring fire and we shared what supper we had with them. The only house near was full of refugees and there was nothing for it but to sleep in the open in the snow. We sat round the camp-fire, and though roasted in front, and frozen behind, we managed to get a few hours' sleep. We took the road at dawn. It was snowing hard, and perishingly cold, and we started with considerable misgivings.

We were now far into the pass, and there could be no turning back. And a big snowstorm during the march through the pass would in all probability have meant the death of thousands, but luckily the snow only lasted for an hour or two. During this part of the Retreat we were often helped by the Albanian peasants, who had posted themselves where they knew their help would be needed with the horses. One would take the pony's

200

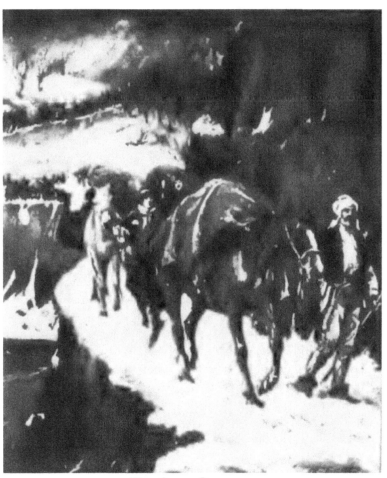

THE GREAT RETREAT

head, and the other the tail, and all three would then slide and slither down the icy descent in the cleverest fashion.

By this time our food-supply was running out, and we were passing through a country where food even in times of peace, is never plentiful. During this part of the march I fear we often forgot Serbia, and the tragedy and death that was going on around us. Our only thoughts were of food, and our talk was of food, and to recall any delicacy would bring our hearts to our mouths. The march through this pass occupied four days in all, and was by far the most trying part of the journey. On the evening of the fourth day we reached more open country. We were now nearing Andrievitza, and the lights of the town were the most cheering sight we had seen for many day.

At Andrievitza we obtained quarters at one of the inns, and here we decided to remain for a day to rest, and try to but provisions. Nothing could be had in the inn, and the shops were mostly closed because there was nothing to sell, but after a long search I managed to buy a sheep, and we were supplied with black bread by the authorities. I borrowed a huge pot from the inn-keeper, and, along with a brother Scot and a Russian medical student, spent the day cooking. I have heard it said that cooks rarely enjoy the meals they prepare—nothing could be more absurd—the soup we made from the sheep was the finest ever made in the Balkan Peninsula.

We expected motor-wagons to take us to Podgoritza, but floods and broken bridges made this impossible. We were feeling fitter after a day's rest, and once more set out at dawn the following morning. A thaw has set in, and the roads were many inches deep in slush and snow. A steep ascent lay before us, and night had fallen before we reached the summit, over 7000 feet above the sea level, the highest point on our trek. From here the road descended sharply, and the ponies they seemed to know the worst was over and assumed quite a rattling pace. We had sent our interpreter on ahead, and to our delight a voice in the darkness hailed us with news of quarters at a Montenegrin inn about a mile beyond. It was not much of an inn, even as inns go in that poor country, and to our way of thinking it was full before we arrived. We cooked our supper at a fire in the middle of one of the three rooms curled up on the floor, and soon fell asleep.

This was the climax of our trek; by another day we were in a different climate, and had left the snow behind. We had still to reach Podgoritza and Scutari The motor-wagons which had been promised us were not forthcoming, so twice again we had to foot it before we saw the Adriatic and San Giovanni di Medua. Provision ships were expected to be waiting there, but when we arrived, the rumour we had heard on the way about Austrian submarines having shelled the port and shipping proved only too true. The wrecks were lying off the shore with the provisions still aboard. The people at San Giovanni were salving what they could, and we lived for several days on bread made from flour reclaimed from the sea.

After camping for three days on the shore, an Italian ship arrived unexpectedly, and the captain arranged to carry the refugees to Italy. The Austrian submarines which had sunk the provision ships were said to be lying in wait outside, but towards midnight the captain decided to risk it, and accompanied by two destroyers we slipped into the night. The next morning we arrived at Brindisi. and our troubles were at an end. We had been part of the Great Retreat for nearly seven weeks. Everyone in my party did well, especially the women, who throughout showed splendid courage and endurance.

Our other party of women under Dr. McGregor, after their retreat from Mladanovatz to Kraguievatz, were sent to Kraljevo, whence via Rashka they went to Mitrovitza, there joining the retreating army. It was just after leaving Rashka that the accident occurred in which one of our finest nurses, Mrs. Toughill, was killed. The car in which she and other nurses were, when passing a huge motor-lorry, went too near the crumbling edge of the road and was capsized over the steep cliff. Mrs. Toughill met with injuries which resulted in her death on the following Sunday, 14th November. From Fortier Jones' book, *With Serbia into Exile*, we get a description of the valley where Rashka lies, and of the very road crawling along the high cliffs where the sad accident occurred:

> The valley of the Ibar is one of the wildest and most beautiful in the world, but in that three days' march we came to regard it as monotonous beyond endurance. Twenty or thirty miles of it out of Rashka surpasses the far-famed Gorges des Loups. The road that twists along the tortuous, shelving cliffs that form its

ranks is as marvellous as the Route des Alpes and as beautiful as any Corniche road must be. Also it is just about as bad as a road could be and still remain a road. Rashka lies in a narrow plain at a widened part of the valley. The road leads out along this plain for a little way, then follows the rapidly rising banks, first on their crest, and later, when they tower to extraordinary heights, is cut from the living rock midway up their sides. With the rising of the banks the valley narrows to a gorge, so that it is like a great funnel, in the widespread mouth of which lies Rashka. Converging at this place, the refugee throngs from most of northern Serbia flowed through this gigantic funnel.

Mention is made of Caroline Toughill, and of all the women who died "on active service" in connection with the S.W.H., in another chapter, but the account in Dr. McGregor's words of the touching-burial-service may well find a place here.

We decided to bury her in a little graveyard on the top of some low hills to the left of the road, on which a tiny hamlet of wattle huts was placed. We climbed up beyond the village and found on the summit of the hill a handful of graves cut into the very rock, and clustering round a little Christian church no more than 20 feet square. Some people in the camp found moss and berries, and a wreath was made. A cross of wood was made by the Serbian surgeon himself, and at three o'clock in the afternoon two priests of the Greek Church came to assist in the religious ceremony. All the officers, soldiers, and prisoners gathered round, and the priest read prayers and made an oration in Serbian in her honour. At the end of this he hailed her as she lay there in the rough soldier's coffin, 'Salve, Carolina' and all the soldiers round about cried. 'Salve, Carolina.' I then read the first part of the burial-service, and then the coffin was carried by relays of soldiers up the steep hill, and there we left her.

Shortly before the accident, Mrs. Toughill had said to one of the nurses with whom she was travelling, "Oh, to be allowed to rest for ever on such a hill and to be alone with God." Dr. McGregor's party and Mr. Smith's met later on and arrived together in England towards the end of December

It is impossible to think of the Great Retreat without calling to the memory the 23,000 Serbian boys who met their fate on that cruel march. To save them from being captured by the enemy 30,000 of the boys of Serbia were ordered out of the country. They made part of the great exodus of their nation. They were young boys from twelve to eighteen years, and they were unable to stand the cold, the hunger, and the physical misery of that march. Fifteen thousand died in the mountains, "and those who saw the ships and the sea had nothing human left of them but their eyes."

> The Italians at Avallona had no hospital accommodation for 15,000. . . . They had the boys encamped in the open country close to a river, and gave them all the food they could spare— army biscuits and bully beef. . . . By the time that the ships to convey them to Corfu arrived the 15,000 had been reduced to 9000. About 2000 more boys died during the twenty-four hours' journey between Avallona and Vido, and thus only 7000 reached the encampment in the grove of orange and olive trees by the sea on the island of Vido.[1]

In the story of another unit of the S.W.H. working in the island of Corsica we pick up again the thread of the lives of some of these 7000 boys, and rejoice that once again, along with other societies, the Scottish Women are to be found "where the need is greatest." A Serbian writer says:

> If the skies were all paper and the sea were all ink we could not even then write the sorrows of our country.

---

1. *With Serbia into Exile.*

CHAPTER 5

Dr. Inglis and Dr. Hollway
at Krushevatz

We have watched Dr. Soltan and her nurses at work in the typhus wards. We have followed Dr. Alice Hutchison's Unit from the day it left Cardiff. We have trekked with the women through the blinding snow across the plain of Kosovo, from town to town we have walked with them, and we have shared with them the horrors of the narrow passes through the Albanian mountains. We have wondered at their fortitude and all their powers of endurance. One writer, speaking of the Englishwomen with whom he made the trek says:

> They were the heroines of the Serbian tragedy, and they realised it not at all.

The women in his particular party did not include any of the Scottish Women, but that does not preclude our claiming the same praise for them. We have now to re-enter Serbia and live through those winter months, from November 1915 to February 1916, with the women left behind in Krushevatz.

Fortier Jones says:

> Krushevatz was the sort of picture which, having once been seen, changes forever the aspect of life. If I were asked to give the death of Serbia in a few sentences. I should tell of a tearless woman beside the shreds of her little boy, struck down by an aeroplane bomb, for 'moral effect;' of old men and young men, old women and young women, boys and girls, starving hopelessly in a frozen wilderness; of the Serbian Army groping and staggering into Scutari, *and of the wounded at Krushevatz*. One does not get rid of such pictures. One goes on living with them

long after the events themselves.

It is here in Krushevatz that we find Dr. Inglis and Dr. Hollway with their party of women. The story of their work there is told in Dr. Inglis' own words, and we have also been fortunate in being given permission to publish extracts from a private diary kept by one of the women in the unit.

Scottish Women's Unit,
Serbian Military Hospital,
Krushevatz, 30th November 1915.

Dear Miss Mair,—We are told we may send letters home—open, of course—so this is to tell the committee that Dr. Hollway's Unit and mine are here working in the Serbian Military Hospital. I enclose a list of the people here, so that you may tell their friends. Dr. Hutchison's Unit is at Vrinjatcha Bania. and Dr. McGregor went southward—possibly you may have heard from her. Some of our people also left with Mr. Smith.

I am sure the committee would approve of our work here. We have charge of the 'Magazine' where the overflow patients from the hospital are taken—about 300 wounded (there are 900 altogether). We are working in the dressing-rooms and certain wards in the hospital—and the director has put all the sanitation and laundry work into our hands. We live in the hospital. There are two rooms given to us.

On the whole, we have been extraordinarily well. Matron has had influenza—but it has not spread at all.

I forgot, in, in telling of our work, to say we have also charge of the little infectious diseases hospital under Dr. Botha. Dr. M—— and two sisters live there.

This is just a bare report for the committee. I cannot tell you what our next move will be. At the present the prisoners are being sent through in thousands. They stay in the hospital grounds, and leave their sick and wounded here, and pass on northward.

The committee must not worry about us. We are well and very busy, and doing the work they sent us out to do.—Ever, dear Miss Mair, yours affectionately,

Elsie Maud Inglis.

Before, however, following the fortunes of the women in Krushevatz, we shall trace with interest the life led by Dr. Hutchison and her unit during their time of imprisonment.

> Scottish Women's Hospital, Vrinjatcha Bania,
> Serbia, 20th November 1915.

Dear Miss Mair,[1]—I expect you never got a letter and wire which I sent you from Pojega about a month ago, reporting everything up to date. I can now, of course, only write very briefly, as we can only write open letters. I asked as a favour from Austrian Headquarters that a wire might be sent to London assuring our people that we are all well, and that there is no cause for anxiety. We knew everyone must be very anxious, and longed often to be able to write home and assure you all that we were wonderfully comfortable, in no danger, and although living very simply compared to our life at Valjevo, that we have never suffered hunger as some I know must be doing.

After getting orders to leave Valjevo, we were moved to Pojega, and then, a week later, down the line to this place. We managed, in spite of a very hurried packing, to bring everything away from Valjevo except the disinfector and our wooden flooring. but during the travelling about we got separated from some of our belongings.

I should like to say that we have not the smallest thing to complain of in our treatment. The difficulty in getting commodities we share with others. Owing to the wish of the Serbian Red Cross to protect the units, five are unfortunately together here, with a very insufficient amount of work. We are now, however to be moved down the line, and will have ample work for which I am glad. In the meantime there has been no proposal to send the units home. Should such a proposal be made, each member will, of course, be left free to do as she likes. Personally, I should prefer to stay on, as I cannot help feeling that before the winter is over there may be great need for medical help. You will understand that I cannot discuss the question further.

For over five weeks we have had no letter or news of any kind from the outside world. That is the most trying thing of all to bear. Everybody has kept in wonderfully good spirits, and it didn't seem to occur to any of us to be afraid. We were more concerned over our inability to battle with Serbian mud! The unit, I am glad to say, has kept well.

---

1. Letter from Dr. Hutchison written after the retreat from Valjevo.

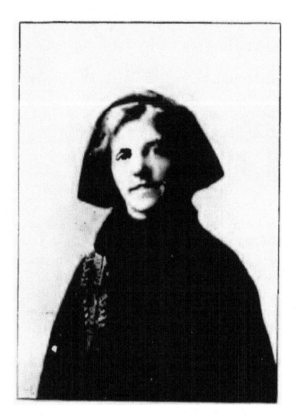

DR. ALICE HUTCHISON

The unit has been loyal, and I have not had many difficulties in our own circle to contend with. I feel it is very unsatisfactory writing in this disjointed way, but I am most anxious to put in nothing which would prevent the letter from going through.

As there is practically nothing private in the letter I should be grateful if you could let it be used for my friends. One could write much of great interest, but that must be kept back. Its strange to know nothing whatever about anything outside this town.

My kindest regards to the committee and to yourself.—Yours very sincerely,   A. M. Hutchison.

You will find out how to communicate with us.

The story of the Valjevo Unit, after the evacuation of their hospital and during the time they were prisoners in the hands of the Austrians, makes good reading because of the unfailing courage and resourcefulness of their "little General," the name the patients in Valjevo gave Dr. Hutchison. No privilege could be got for the women in her charge was unclaimed, nor any bad treatment that could be averted allowed to continue if "the little General," waving the Geneva Convention in the face of the Austrians, could obtain what was necessary. She once sadly remarked, "The Austrians do not seem ever to have heard of the Geneva Convention!" In the beginning of October the unit was hurriedly moved from Valjevo to Pojega, taking their equipment with them. Here they were to form a base hospital, but they had hardly got into working order, when they were again moved to Vrinjatcha Bania, which was reached on 29th October, where they were given a hospital of a hundred beds.

On 10th November the enemy took possession of the town. They behaved well, and the Scottish women were allowed to carry on their work In the end of the month, however, the unit was ordered to Krushevatz, where Dr. Inglis was, ostensibly to work in a hospital there. They were not, however, allowed to take their equipment, which was seized by the enemy for use in their hospitals. But Dr. Hutchison refused to give it up until she obtained a receipt for it, in order that it might be paid for after the war, according to the provisions of the Geneva Convention. At Krushevatz the only complaint made by the women was, that in the hotel where they were billeted the officers' table was always served first, with the result that there was seldom enough food for the women in the background!

During my[2] peregrinations over the town I came on Dr. Inglis and her unit. If I had up till then felt that we in no way merited the title of 'the heroic band of women,' I came away from Dr. Inglis' hospital feeling that they *had* earned it. Picture over twenty people—including the head of the hospital-dining and sleeping and eating and washing in one room;[3] picture all their equipment gone, and them looking after Serbs in the best way they could in hospital corridors. They were, however, wearing no air of martyrdom.

On 4th December they were again moved, and in a few days arrived at Kevavara, in the plains of Hungary, where they stayed nearly three months. The food at first was not good:

"I found it was exactly the same as the rations served out to the Russians and Italians who were prisoners, so I made a protest pointing out that doctors were entitled to officer' treatment under the Geneva Convention. After this we got better bread, and fresh meat sometimes."

During all the weary weeks at Kevavara the spirits of the women never failed. They played rounders sometimes in the little yard behind the house where they lived. They enjoyed long walks, though the Austrian guard who had to accompany them did not.

"After one expedition our guard got so tired that he complained to the captain, though we had only been about six or eight miles. He reported that it would not be so bad if we would only walk, but we 'flew like geese over the mud.'"

"Three armed men were on guard day and night in the passage, and at first were very surly, but gradually their behaviour improved, till at last they were quite friendly. We used to borrow their uniforms for, the charades and *tableaux* which we got up to pass the evenings, and sometimes they took part in these themselves, but not when we represented the *Kaiser* or Emperor Joseph."

On Christmas, Day we had quite a jolly time, with a Christmas tree and a first-rate dinner. We went out and got some live geese from the market, which were killed and cooked, and we had all kinds of cakes, and even butter—at five shillings a pound! In

---

2. Quotation from Dr. Hutchison's report.
3. Later on Dr. Hutchison herself had to suffer the same hardships, her party of thirty-two being entirely confined to two small rooms during her three months' stay in Kevavara.

the evening we sang carols and drank toasts. We even ventured for the first time to sing 'God Save the King' under our breath. After this we sang it every night, and it cheered us up wonderfully. We had our British flag with us to too. I wound it round my body, under my clothes, when we evacuated our hospital, so that it should not be trampled upon and insulted.

On 4th February they were taken to Budapest, and from there to Vienna, where their troubles were practically at an end. On their arrival in Switzerland, as they crossed the border, they waved the precious flag out of the windows and shouted, "God Save the King."

On her return home. Dr. Inglis wrote an account of their work in Krushevatz for the Englishwoman of June 1916. The following extracts are taken from that articles:

The units left at Krushevatz, however, were the fortunate units. To them fell the honour of caring for the Serbian wounded through the first three tragic months of the foreign occupation. At first they worked on two parties: the one in the Girls' School, which was arranged on the lines of the hospital at Kraguievatz, with the equipment brought from there; and the other at the Serbian Military Hospital.—the Czar Lazar Hospital,—where they were given charges of the annexe formed in the storehouses. The hospital at the Girls' School had a short, if brilliant. career, for it was seized with all its equipment, by the Germans two days after their entry. 'Of course they took it,' said our Serbian Director. 'You had made it so beautiful.'

After the loss of the Girls' School both units worked at the Czar Lazar until it was evacuated on the 9th of February.

'The German occupation of Krushevatz was heralded in proper form by bombardment. The Serbs blew up a railway bridge, which attracted their fire, and they threw three bombs and several shells into the town. We fell that we had had our baptism of fire.

Their entry next morning, 7th November, was almost in the form of an anticlimax. We turned into the principal street to find a German regiment lined up there. The best of the Serbs had left, while flags were hanging out of most of the occupied house, and Krushevatz was taken. . . .

The Czar Lazar Hospital was in a building designed for the barracks, and could have held comfortably four hundred beds. In the grounds were two small buildings, intended as the hospital in connection with the barracks, two big stores, or magazines, as we always called them, and numerous outhouses. When we went up there, there were nine hundred patients, three hundred of them in the magazine under Dr. Hollway. During the greatest pressure the numbers rose to one thousand two hundred. Patients were placed in the corridors—at first one man to one bed, but later two beds together and three men in them. Then there were no more bedsteads; mattresses were placed on the floors. We filled up the outhouses. The magazine in full blast was a sight, once seen, never to be forgotten.

The ground flat had an uneven earthen floor, not the place one would choose to nurse surgical patients. Dr. Corbett and Dr. Scott—the latter had come home from New Zealand 'to do her bit'—in charge. But upstairs in Dr. Hollway's domain, the patients occupied the shelving which ran the whole length of the building in four rows. There were three tiers, the slightly wounded men in the highest tier. The time of day to see the magazine at its best—or rather at its worst—was in the gloaming, when two or three feeble oil lamps shed an uncertain light over the scene, and the tin bowls clattered and rattled as the evening ration of beans was given out, and the men swarmed up and down the poles of their shelves, chattering as Serbs will chatter. The sisters called the place the 'Zoo,' the only name to describe it.

We could not take away the men's uniforms either in the magazines or corridors, for the weather was bitterly cold, and there was already a shortage of fuel. This fact, taken with the overcrowding and the condition of the men,—fatigued, depressed, and underfed,—made the possibility of an outbreak of typhus a very real danger. At the request of the director of the hospital, Major Nicolitch, we opened a small building in the grounds as an infectious diseases hospital, and he appealed to the Austrians for the use of another building to relieve overcrowding, 'There is no other building,' was the answer, though all the time the upper storey of the prefecture was empty (the lower one was used as a store for Red Cross equipment, which they had taken from us without receipts), and the fact was brought to their notice.

But we soon realised that no help was to be expected from that quarter, and that we must help ourselves. So we improvised a bathroom in the corner of the magazine, took over all the bathing arrangements for the hospital, set the two French disinfectors going, with the help of a Russian, and one of ourselves, who was something of a mechanic and last and most important of all, we took over the laundry, and the hospital got clean linen We worked round the hospital, bathing and disinfecting every five days. In this connection we must always remember Sister Strange's name, who took over this very necessary if uninteresting work, from the point of view of a fully trained nurse, and carried it through triumphantly. We had not a single case of typhus .

Only two cases of typhus appeared in our little infectious diseases hospital, and they were both from among the civilian population. We heard that there were a great many cases in the Austrian Army.

Later the director made over to us the whole downstairs flat of the hospital, with the room for dressings and the medical ward, as well as the little hospital for infectious cases, the magazine. the laundry, the sanitation. There was one bit of work which we were offered and refused to take—the care of women suffering from venereal disease. It was very difficult to refuse, with our modern vision of the solidarity of womanhood, but the hospital was not opened for the safety of the women but for the protection of the German Army. To have taken over that work would have been to encourage vice and that we could not do.

Perhaps the most important department was the sanitation. We had not an expert amongst us; but when Dr. Hutchison's Unit passed through. her Sanitary Inspector, Miss Gordon, came up to inspect us, and was pleased with the result.

When we arrived, that hospital compound was a truly terrible place—the sights and smells beyond description. We dug into the ground the rubbish, emptied the overflowing cesspools. built incinerators, and cleaned, and cleaned, and cleaned. That is a Briton's job all over the world, and our three untrained British orderlies took to it like ducks to water. It was not the pleasantest or easiest work in the world; but they did it, and did it magnificently. Miss W—— especially developed wonderful powers of command—managed her men, fed them, clothed them, and left that hospital compound not, it is true, exactly like an English park, but at least clean.

The prisoners taken in the south were brought through Krushevatz on their way to the Concentration Camps in Hungary—one day as many as three thousand. We had seen these men all through the summer just beyond our camps at Mladanovatz and Valjevo with their heads held high, and conscious of the good work they had done for the Allies in driving back the Austrian 'punitive expedition.' They used to say to us with such childlike pride, 'We are the only ones who, so far, have beaten our enemy.' They came back to us broken and dispirited men, over-fatigued, and dirty, and underfed. They were turned into the hospital grounds, given their scanty ration of beans with a little meat and half a loaf of bread for twenty-four hours.

For some weeks they got only quarter of a loaf—one loaf among four men. Their camp-fires flickered fitfully through the long, bitter cold nights. Every scrap of wood in the enclosure was torn up: the doors and windows from the buildings wrecked by the first bombardment; the little foot-bridge over the drains; the trees hacked down. One night the scene might have been the retreat from Moscow. The ground was white with snow, a fine blizzard was blowing, almost blotting out in the distance the crouching figures of the men as they sat in their ragged uniforms round the fires. . . .

There was shortage of food even while we were there. Remember what a hospital diet usually is, and then remember that we had to feed our patients on beans and a scanty allowance of meat—which was not always good—half a loaf of bread a day for each man, and some weak tea. One day the director got five hundred eggs, but they were seized at the hospital gates by the Austrians. There was rice in the stores, and we had some sacks too and we boiled it up with condensed milk and made 'sutlyage,' which added something to the diet, but when sugar failed, as it did eventually, half the good of this addition failed also. Our administrator, Mrs. Haverfield, scoured the country for milk and eggs, and we bought what we could with the Scottish funds, but it was not enough.

These months at Krushevatz were a strange mixture of sorrow and happiness. Was the country really so very beautiful, or was it the contrast to all the misery that made it evident? There was a curious exhilaration in working for those grateful, patient men, and in helping the director, so loyal to his country, and so conscientious in his work, to bring order out of chaos and yet the unhappiness in the Serbian houses, and the physical wretchedness of those cold, hungry prisoners, lay always like a dead weight on our spirits. Never shall we forget the beauty at the sunrises or the glory of the sunsets with clear, cold, sunlight days between, and the wonderful starlight nights.

But we shall never forget 'the Zoo' either, or the groans outside when we hid our heads in the blankets to shut out the sound. Nor shall we ever forget the cheeriness or trustfulness of all that hospital, and especially of the officers' ward. We got no news, and we made it a point of honour not to believe a word of the German telegrams posted up in the town. So we lived on rumour, and what rumour! The English at Skoplje, the Italians at Pojega, and the Russians over the Carpathians—we could not believe that Serbia had been sacrificed for nothing. We were convinced it was some deep-laid scheme for weakening the other fronts, and so it was quite natural to hear that the British had taken Belgium and the French were in Metz.

When we reached Zurich and found everything much the same as when we disappeared into the silence, our hearts were sick for the people we left behind us still waiting and trusting.

At last, on the 9th of February, our hospital was emptied. The chronic invalids had been 'put on commission' and sent to their homes. The vast majority of the men had been removed to Hungary, and the few remaining, badly wounded men who would not be fit for months, taken over to the Austrian hospitals.

On the 11th we were sent north under an Austrian guard with fixed bayonets. Great care was taken that we should not communicate with anyone *en route*. At Belgrade, however, we were put into a waiting-room for the night, and after we had crept into our sleeping-bags we were suddenly roused to speak to a Serbian woman. The kindly Austrian officer in charge of us said she was the wife of a Serbian officer in Krushevatz, and that if we would use only German we might speak to her. She wanted news of her husband. We were able to reassure her. He was getting better—he was in the gymnasium. '*Vrylo dobra*' ('Very well'), she said, holding both our hands. '*Vrylo, vrylo dobra,*' we said, looking apprehensively at the officer. But he only laughed.

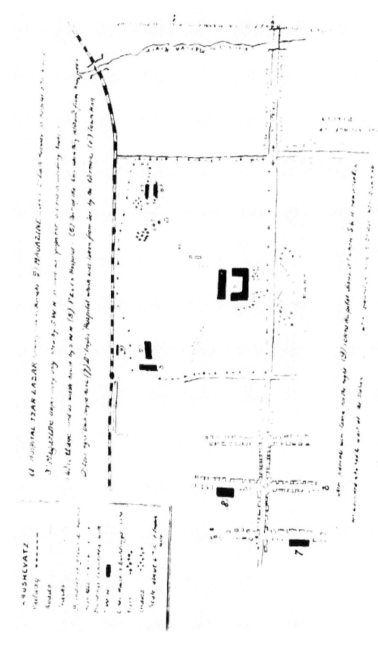

PLAN OF THE CZAR LAZAR HOSPITAL AND GROUNDS

Probably his Serbian, too, was equal to that.

That was the last Serbian we spoke to in Serbia, and we left her a little happier.

And thus we came to Vienna, where the American Embassy took us over. When we thanked one of the secretaries for all the infinite trouble they had taken, he answered in truly American phrase: 'Well, I cannot say it has been any trouble. But it has taken some doing.'

From Vienna we went to Bludenz, where, thanks to 'military reasons,' we had eight days' delightful rest; and then to Zurich.

A plan of the Czar Lazar Hospital and its grounds is given, because it is felt that the scene of the wonderful work done by the Scottish Women through those winter months is full of interest, a work which has been one of the strongest factors in binding our little Ally with us in bonds of friendship.

Further, those who know her best feel that it was here, going in spirit with her beloved Serbs through their time of extremest woe, that Dr. Inglis' "heart broke," and the "beginning of the end" came upon her. . . .

But we cannot end on this note. For Serbia we know, that "sunset in the West is sunrise in the East." And as regards the Scottish Women we are glad to hear of them "playing" in the station at Belgrade, where they were kept waiting several hours, seeing how long they could walk along a rail of the railway lines without slipping off! Also we rejoice in the thought of their first breakfast at Vienna when told by Dr. Inglis that they were to eat as much as they wanted and the unit would pay, they each had "plates and plates of ham and eggs, and cups and cups of coffee."

LETTER FROM M. PACHITCH, PRIME MINISTER OF SERBIA,

Claridge's Hotel,
London, 4th April 1916.

To the President of the Executive Committee of the Scottish Women's Hospitals for Foreign Service.

Dear Madam.—Our Minister in London, Monsieur Boschko-vitch, informs me that Drs. E. Inglis and Hutchison, together with the members of their representative units, have recently returned from Serbia, where they had remained as long as they could, taking care of our wounded soldiers.

In the name of His Royal Highness the Crown Prince, in the

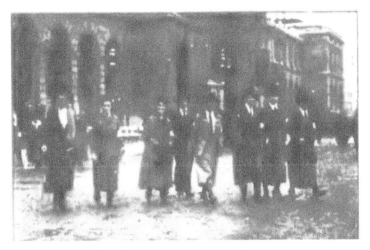

DR. INGLIS AND PARTY AT ZURICH

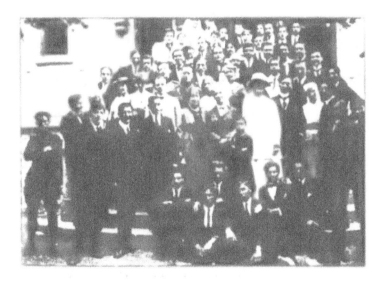

GROUP OF PATIENTS AT SALLANCHES

name of the Serbian Government and of the whole Serbian nation, I have the honour to convey through you the expressions of our highest gratitude to the noble daughters of the great British nation who have risked their lives and sacrificed their freedom for the health and the good of the Serbian soldier and the Serbian people.

I avail myself of this opportunity to tell you how much we appreciate the help rendered to Serbia by the Scottish Women's Association, who sent so many and so splendidly organised hospitals to our country, and who are still continuing to help our people as much as they can.

The Serbian nation will never forget what the Scottish Women have done for them.—Yours very sincerely,

    (Sgd.)   Prime Minister of Serbia,

                              Nik. P. Pachitch.

By Miss Edith Palliser.

CHAPTER 1

Mejidia

In the month of July 1916 the Serbian Minister in London, M. Boskovitch, asked Dr. Inglis if the Scottish Women's Hospitals would be willing to supply one or more of four field hospitals for service with the Serb Division in Russia. As soon as this request was made known to the Scottish Women's Hospitals by Dr. Inglis, the London Units Committee of the Scottish Women's Hospitals offered to equip and maintain two of these field hospitals, with a motor transport attached to them. At the time, Dr. Inglis was busy in making preparations to take out a Unit to the Serbian Army in Salonika, but when she found that these Serbs in Russia were in very great need of medical relief she decided to accept the offer to take charge of the Field Hospitals and Transport Section and go to Russia.

That a clear understanding and appreciation of subsequent events affecting the relations between Dr. Inglis and the Serb Division may be reached, a brief account of its genesis must be given here.

The division consisted mainly of Serbo-Croats and Slovenes, that is. Serbs who, as subjects of Austria-Hungary, were obliged to serve in the Austrian Army. Nearly all of these men had been taken prisoners by the Russians or, perhaps more correctly, had voluntarily surrendered to the Russians rather than fight for the enemies of their conationals. In May, 1915 a considerable number of these Austro-Serbs volunteered for service with the Serbian Army, and by arrangement with the Russian Government, who gave them their freedom, they were transported to Serbia. After the entry of Bulgaria into the war it was no longer possible to send them to Serbia, and 2000 were left behind at Odessa.

The number of these volunteers increased, however, to such an

extent that, by permission of the Serbian Government, Serbian officers from Corfu were sent over to organise them into a military unit
for service with the Russian Army. By May 1916, a first division was
formed under the command of the Serb colonel, Colonel Hadjitch,
and later a second division under General Zivkovitch. It was to the
first division that the Field Hospitals and Transport were to be attached.

The unit mustered at Liverpool on the 29th of August, and left for
Archangel on the following day. It consisted of a personnel of seventy-
five, with three doctors, in charge of Dr. Elsie Inglis, C.M.O.

In a letter, Dr. Inglis gave an account of the voyage to Archangel,
which was "a most pleasant one and very restful."

> This is a very steady little boat, and we have had very calm
> weather after the first day, when we pitched and tossed a good
> deal. The majority of the unit collapsed, but reappeared none
> the worse, and bustling with energy! The British girl is a very
> delightful creature.
>
> Some of them were really too funny the day of the alarm for
> boat drill quite indignant that there was no submarine there.
> We did sight a submarine early one morning, but she took no
> notice of us, so we took none of her. She was very big, possibly
> the *Deutschland*.

They reached Archangel on the 10th of September, and heard that
their destination was Odessa. From the moment of their landing in
Russia, and throughout their journey south, the unit met with a most
cordial welcome. Dr. Inglis in her letters repeatedly refers to the extraordinary kindness shown them both by the Russian officials and
their own countrymen. A magnificent reception was given to the unit
on their arrival at Odessa on the 21st of September. The governor of
the town, the head of the medical department of the Russian Army,
the British Consul and Mrs. Bagge, and numerous Russian officials
met them at the station. Twenty Serb officers were also present, lined
up to salute them.

The news that greeted Dr. Inglis was grave. General Zivkovitch
informed her that the first division was in action and had suffered
heavily. Later, a full account of the battle showed that the Serb Division had gone into the fight 14,000 strong, they were in the centre,
with the Roumanians on the left and the Russians on the right. The
Roumanians and Russians broke, and the Serbs, who had fought for

twenty-four hours on two fronts, came out with only 4000 men.

General Zivkovitch was at first inclined to keep the hospital at Odessa to take charge of 1000 wounded Serbs, and to send the transport immediately to the front. Dr. Inglis expressed her willingness to carry out his wishes, but explained that if her hospital were separated from its transport it would become practically stationary, and it was not equipped for this. General Zivkovitch saw the reasonableness of these representations and it was decided that the unit should go on to the front. He asked Dr. Inglis to make arrangements meanwhile for the care of the wounded Serbs in the town. This she gladly consented to do, and she was successful in obtaining from the Russian authorities a building admirably suited for a hospital. In this task Dr. Inglis had the invaluable aid of the British Consul. Mr. Bagge, who introduced her to the leading Russian authorities, and was unsparing in his efforts to render her assistance in every way.

The days of waiting at Odessa were enlivened by constant festivities. It was not. indeed, possible for the unit to accept the cordial invitations showered upon them. Chief among these events were the Serb Mess dinner and the gala performance at the Opera House. At the Serb Mess, Dr. Inglis and her party received a rousing welcome. As they entered the room the two hundred officers rose and greeted them with cheers which were all but deafening. General Zivkovitch himself was present part of the time, and the guests were entertained by songs and dances. All the national anthems were sung, including the Croatian and Czech national airs.

Of the gala performance at the opera Dr. Inglis gives the following account:

> The mayor of the town sent us tickets for the performance at the opera. Fourteen boxes were put at our disposal, sufficient to accommodate everybody. After the second act the grand duchess[1] intimated that she wished to inspect the whole unit, and we were accordingly drawn up in the corridor. The consul presented me to her, and then I presented the officers. She walked down the whole row, speaking to all the members. . . . When we returned to our seats the orchestra played the British National Anthem three times, and the third time the unit took up the air and sang. The whole audience rose, turned towards us, cheering and waving handkerchiefs. We all felt so touched. It is a great

---

1. Olga Petrovna, an aunt of the *Czar*.

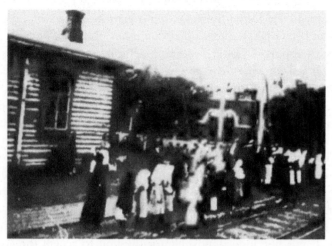

On the way to Odessa

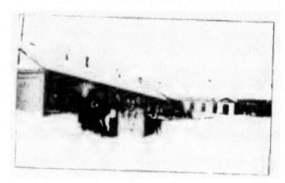

The hospital at Mejidia

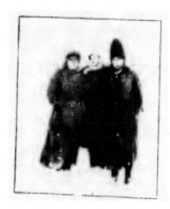

Winter at Mejidia

thing to feel that we are going on to our work with so much enthusiasm behind us.[2]

On Monday, the 25th of September, the unit left Odessa for Reni *en route* to Czernavoda, where Dr Inglis was to receive her instructions. This journey, which in ordinary times was a matter of some five or six hours occupied four days and three nights. The long delays were the more trying to all, haunted as they were by the thought of how urgently they were needed. It was quite usual to wait two hours for every half-hour travelled, and the rate of progress was so slow that some members of the unit would jump out and run alongside the train.

We meandered quietly through the country. We went into the villages and saw the people and the churches while we waited at the stations. A great many of the unit basked in the sunshine on the open trucks which carried the motors. At one village where some of us came in for a service, it being a feast day, the priest was reading the New Testament lesson, and when he had ended he said. 'Let us pray for the English sisters who have come to help us.' At another village the priest came in and blessed our food. The children were always most friendly. In one place, a little Jewish girl, in their funny German dialect, told us she knew all about England; she had learnt about it at school and England was 'little, little'—putting her forefinger and thumb together—and Russia was big 'like that'—throwing her arms wide. The Russian officials were very kind, and as helpful as they could be, but at last in despair I wired back to Odessa to say we must have a Russian officer on our train. We wondered very much if the telegram got through, but we certainly got on more quickly after that, and we heard later that the telegram did arrive.[3]

From Reni the "Greys" as the Hospital Staff were called (to distinguish them from the Transport, who wore khaki and were called the "Buffs"), went by steam-launch down the Danube to Czernavoda. There they were met by an Irishman, an officer in the Russian Army, who, Dr. Inglis said, "spoke Russian like a Russian, French like a Frenchman, and English like an Irishman, not to mention Spanish. Italian, German, Hindu, and a few other odds and ends." This officer's name was

---

2.& 3 Dr. Inglis' report.

Bryson, and he was most helpful in seeing them and the equipment on to the train for Mejidia. There they arrived at eleven at night and slept in the train, no arrangements having been made for them. The Transport section had a more uncomfortable experience. The cars and lorries had to be taken down to Czernavoda in two barges, and there was no accommodation for the drivers. They lived, slept, and ate where they could find room on the iron decks, without any shelter.

They were told they would arrive in Czernavoda in a few hours, but the few hours lengthened out to a night and a day. On landing at Czernavoda at night they found the place deserted: all the civilians had evacuated the town. There was no food, and, to make matters worse, the rain came down in torrents and the wind was blowing half a gale.

The drivers stayed by their cars all night, taking turns at sentry-go. At daylight, preparations were made to leave:

> So in streaming rain and seas of mud we made a start. After about ten kilometres the stone road came to an end, and there we saw, stuck, in the mud in every kind of attitude of helplessness, several Russian lorries that had been in the barges next to us on the journey up, and had gone off in the inky darkness the previous evening with much noise and bluster.
>
> The road having come to an end, we had to go along a track through fields. Here began many strenuous hours of real labour. There was a specially steep pitch to be surmounted, the soft surface preventing the wheels getting any grip, but with rope around the rear wheels and much pushing and heaving, all were got up including the big lorries. On arriving at Mejidia we discovered we had come the wrong way in spite of our guide. The distance covered was only fifteen miles, but it took eight hours to reach Mejidia! [4]

The day after the hospitals arrived at Mejidia Dr. Inglis saw Colonel Hadjitch at the Serb Headquarters at Bulbul Mic, and they decided to take a barrack offered by the head of the Russian Medical Department and open a hospital at Mejidia, the cars to run out to Bulbul Mic, about ten miles, to bring in patients.

Dr. Inglis wrote:

> It was no good in the world talking about regular Field Hospitals to them, until they had tried our mettle. The ordinary male

---

4. Mrs Haverfield's report.

disbelief in our capacity cannot be argued away; it can only be worked away.

It was not long before the Serb and Russian authorities received proof of the capacity of the unit for hard work, and of their powers of endurance under the strain and stress of war conditions.

The same day, 2nd October, the operations of cleaning and white-washing the barrack were begun. Half the equipment was unloaded and sent up to the hospital and for its better security. Dr. Potter and Dr. Corbett made it their bed for the night.

That evening, after we were all in bed, a Russian officer came to ask if we were ready for wounded. A message was sent down saying 'No.' Then the question came up, 'When will you be ready?' and I sent back the answer. 'Tomorrow evening.' The unit took it with the greatest calmness; only Mrs. Haverfield murmured from her bed. 'I wonder you did not say tonight!'[5]

The hospital stood on the top of a hill overlooking Mejidia. On the hill were other barracks, one occupied by the Russian Red Cross and another by the 2nd Serb Lazarette, to which the unit was attached.

The barrack had two storeys: on each storey was a long room divided down the middle by a brick partition which did not reach up to the ceiling, so there was a thorough draught. At either end were three or four small rooms: office, bathroom, and disinfecting room. For the first five days the unit camped in the top room—seventy-five in one room—an arrangement which did not make for comfort, especially as work had to be carried on at full pressure during those days; but everyone bore the discomfort cheerfully.

No patients arrived that night (Tuesday), but the next morn-ing the cars were ordered out, and at once the wounded began to pour in. We bathed them all and dressed most (but the first dressings were excellently done), and had done four necessary operations by 3 o'clock the next morning. We had taken in 102 patients, two of whom died almost immediately, and we were full. The cars had been running steadily both to the hospital and the station until after 10, when Mrs. Haverfield ordered the chauffeurs to bed, to start again at 5 a.m. Miss Henderson got no sleep that night, for she insisted on seeing us to bed first and then the transport off at 5. We evacuated almost half our patients

5. Dr. Inglis' report.

alter forty-eight hours' rest and took in more, but we found 100 mattresses in those two rooms too close for proper nursing, so we reduced the number to 75, and decided to pitch our camp for the personnel and take the upstairs floor tor the hospital.

Then Dr. Hartsoff (Head of the Russian Medical Department) asked me to take over another small barrack, and I agreed on condition that he gave me the mattresses. However, before that could be accomplished, orders came in from the Serb Head-quarters to send Hospital 'B' out to Bulbul Mic, so I told Dr. Hartsoff we could not undertake more than one barrack at Mejidia, but I promised 140 beds there, including two rooms for officers.

More than half our patients were Russians. We had two Roua-nians. It was very interesting to see how the attitude of our patients altered as the days went on. Our Serbs, as always, were grateful and trusting but the Russians could not at all under-stand the situation. They were very reluctant to come into the operating-room, and grumbled to the numerous officers who came in and out. One of the officers, quite a boy sent for me and said brusquely that the men were not getting enough food. I thought it time to stop it so I said quite firmly that there was ample food, and that I should like him to remember that we were a Serb hospital and that the diet was arranged on Serb lines; that I was more than willing to take in Russian soldiers, but if they did not like it they need not come.

In quite a different tone he said the Russian soldier always wanted *kasha*, a kind of bean porridge. So I said if that was the only difficulty, *kasha* they should have I remembered what Mrs. Kinnell [6] had said about tea, and increased that in quantity. The Russian sisters in the other barrack kindly allowed their cook to teach ours how to make *kasha*, and I went down to the Rus-sian Headquarters and demanded *kasha*. The dear little Russian sister put her finger on another sore point: 'they do not love open windows.' she said, 'and they do not love to be so clean.'

On these two points we were adamant, and it was very interest-ing to see how human nature accommodated itself. Gradually the faces began to smile, and the inquiring officers used to turn to us and say. 'He says everything is good; the only difficulty is

---

6. Mrs. Kinnell, vice-chairman of the London Committee of the Scottish Women's Hospitals.

the language.' One boy who had his arm amputated said, 'It is so good here I am in no hurry to go back to Russia.' We got a Serb student to come round twice a day and interpret for us. and then a Serb who could speak English and Russian to be orderly in the ward. He liked to be called 'Chris,' and had a strenuous time, night and day, at everybody's call. He was most helpful and willing. [7]

The transport had been attached to the 1st Serb Hospital and had no easy time driving in a strange country with the roads in such a terrible condition. Mrs. Haverfield's description of their work gives a vivid picture of the difficulties encountered. Two places, Equibior and Bulbul Mare, from which they had to bring patients, were about fifteen kilometres from Mejidia station.

The road to Equibior was just a track across endless plains after leaving the main road to Bulbul Mare. Here the usual struggle began to get the cars through the mud. We found the place all smoking, and much battered by shells. We filled up with the wounded, two in each car, and got them safely back.

After a few days of this work we received the order to pitch camp at Bulbul Mic, ten miles from Mejidia, Here enemy aeroplanes visited us daily, dealing death and destruction everywhere, but we all escaped injury. The days were lovely and warm, but the nights were very cold and damp.

Suddenly wounded began to pour in, and we and the hospital worked night and day. Things were not going well at the front, and we were told we might have to evacuate at any moment.

There were a few cases of cholera, and we were asked to keep an ambulance separate from the others in order to take cases to the isolation hospitals. One of the drivers (Ruth Plimsoll) had charge of the particular ambulance, and drove a wounded officer all the way to Czernavoda, accompanied by the doctor. When they arrived there the doctor went to find the right place to deposit his patient—a longer process, and meanwhile bombs suddenly began to fall on all sides. Ruth Plimsoll remained calmly on her seat, and when the doctor returned and the car moved away a bomb fell in the exact spot where the ambulance had been waiting, making a large hole in the ground.

The patient, in spite of his pain, insisted on having Ruth Plim-

7. Dr. Inglis report.

soll's name written down, and told the doctor that if he lived he would see she got a special decoration for the great courage she had shown. Most of our drivers have been in the midst of falling bombs whilst carrying wounded, especially to the station, and all have shown the highest courage and perfect calmness amidst frantic panic on the part of all in the street at the time.[8]

In response to the order from Serb Headquarters, Dr. Chesney was sent to Bulbul Mic to form a Field Hospital (Hospital "B"), and the equipment was sent out in charge of four orderlies.

Dr. Inglis wrote:

That was the first time I realised what a first-rate unit I had. Although Bulbul Mic was only ten miles off they look twenty-four hours to get there. They refused to sleep in the passenger carriage provided for them for fear the equipment waggon should be slipped, so they camped in the waggon. I worried a good deal over their having no food with them, when I heard they had not arrived at Bulul Mic, but they were fed by Serb officers, and arrived smiling saying they 'had had the time of their lives'

Dr. Chesney found on arrival that what was wanted was a clearing station that could be evacuated at an hours notice, so almost all there equipment was sent back. She made a beautiful little camp. All her transport was arranged for by Dr. Stanovitch (medical director of the 1st Serb Lazarette. to which she was attached). She kept only ten of the unit with her, including Miss Henderson (Administrator).

The work at Mejidia, with the exception of a few days lull, went forward steadily from the 3rd of October until the 22nd.

On the 19th the sound of the guns became both more intense and continuous. The raids from enemy aeroplanes over Mejidia averaged about three or four a day, and there were several casualties. At one time a falling bomb killed two soldiers in the courtyard of the hospital.

The first intimation that all was not going well at the front was the news that Dr. Chesney had left Bulbul Mic and fallen back about eight miles, halfway to Mejidia. Then came orders from Colonel Hadjitch. by a special dispatch rider, to remove the bulk of the equipment of the Scottish Women's Hospitals and to keep only what was necessary to carry on the hospital at Mejidia.

---

8. Mrs. Haverfield's report.

From the Russian Headquarters Dr. Inglis had the disquieting information that she must not count on a train for taking the equipment. What was to be done? Forty-five tons of equipment could not be taken by three lorries. Dr. Inglis, never recognising such a word as impossible, went to the commandant at the railway station and explained how precious the equipment was and what its delay and probable loss would entail. Three wagons were then supplied at 1 p m., the equipment was packed, and by 3 a.m. the camp was struck.

While waiting for their train to leave, Miss Bowerman and Miss Brown, who were seated on the platform, saw to their consternation the wagons and the precious equipment disappearing with a refugee train. In a flash they were on their feet and in full flight after the train, which they triumphantly boarded. The wagons, however, were shunted again and again and repeatedly held up, until these resourceful women hit upon the expedient of writing telegrams to British Consuls, which they never intended to send, and inventing a General Popovitch who, they said, would be very angry indeed if the equipment did not get through quickly. This bluff was perfectly successful, so much so that they began to wonder whether a General Popovitch really did exist.

The whole of the unit went to Galatz in charge of Dr. Corbett. Dr. Inglis only kept what was absolutely necessary to carry on the hospital or any other she might have to form, seventeen persons in all.

The station was a curious sight that night. The flight was beginning. A crowd of people was collected at one end with boxes and bundles and children. One little boy was lying on a doorstep asleep, and against the wall, farther on, lay a row of soldiers. On the bench to the right, under the light, was a doctor in his white overall, stretched out sound asleep between the two rushes of work at the station dressing-room; and a Roumanian officer talked to me of Glasgow, where he had once been invited out to dinner—so he had seen the British 'customs.' It was good to feel those British customs were still going quietly on, whatever was happening here—breakfasts coming regularly, hot water for baths, and everything as it should be. It was probably absurd, but it came like a great wave of comfort to feel that Britain was there, quiet, strong, and invincible, behind everything and everybody. [9]

---

9. Dr. Inglis' report.

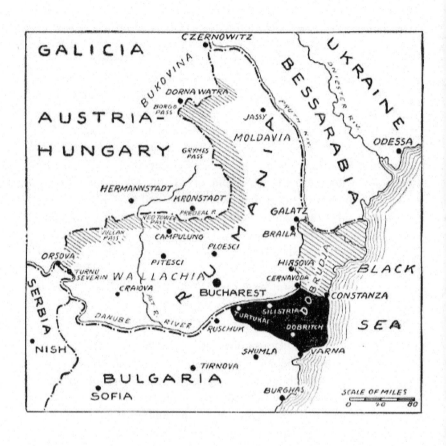

The Retreat From the Dobrudja

On Sunday morning, October the 22nd, Mejidia was practically deserted, except for Dr. Inglis and her party: the Russian hospital had slipped away quietly without any notice to Dr. Inglis of their departure, and scarcely a chimney smoked in the town. The stillness was broken only by the booming of the guns, sounding very near. Dr. Kostitch brought the order at 10 a.m. to evacuate immediately. Every car that could be spared had been sent to Mrs. Haverfield for the wounded and there remained the staff car, one ambulance, and a lorry lent by a young Russian officer. The party set out on their journey that afternoon.

As far as Carlos Premier the run might have been an ordinary one through any country with second-rate roads, at any time. When we turned eastward at Carlos Premier we met the whole stream of refugees from Constanza and the south. One reads of refugees but never could imagine such a sight. The whole road was one continuous stream of carts loaded up with luggage on which were children: men and women tramped along beside them. Every now and again there was a regular cart with boards stretched across measuring from 10 to 12 feet, piled up with household goods—they filled the whole roadway. Against this stream we tried to go, and through it barged cannon and ammunition wagons, and squadrons of cavalry.

Loose foals and dogs ran about everywhere, and when we turned on our headlights the whole thing became unreal—seemed like a well staged piece at the theatre. At one point we came on a flock of sheep, and for a minute we saw only red lights reflected from ours in their eyes—no sheep at all, on foal got quite mesmerised by our lights and danced about in front of them. Suddenly another car loomed out of the darkness, and there were two of our transport girls. Eventually we got into Caromarat, where a room was found for us by a Serb officer. [1]

They all slept very soundly that night on the straw-covered floor, and were joined next morning by Mrs. Haverfield, Miss Henderson, and the rest of the transport.

The party of seven who had become separated from Dr. Inglis on leaving Mejidia landed at Saragea, where they were hospitably cared for by the Russian Headquarters. They sent a message to Dr. Inglis to say they were safe, but completely stranded, as the borrowed Russian lorry had taken its departure. Dr. Inglis went over to their rescue and found them in the verandah of an inn, seated on the equipment, smiling.

Dr. Inglis wrote:

I thought that there might be something in what a Russian woman said to me *apropos* of the great cheerfulness of the unit: 'There is certainly something great in the British character which the continental nations do not possess.' And when I replied 'I don't know, we all have our strong points and our weak ones,' she said 'There is no other nation goes into trouble smiling.'

Hospital "B" with the 1st Serb Lazarette, had been hard at work, dealing with a constant stream of wounded at Bulbul Mic when the order came on 20th October for them to fall back to a little village eight miles to the rear. All the wounded had then been sent to Mejidia. The next day, 21st October, at 5 p.m., they started off, a party of ten, each perched on the top of a pile of equipment in the wagons provided for them by the 1st Serb Hospital, their destination unknown. On the 23rd they came across Dr. Inglis in the darkness, seated in her car, where she was waiting for the light of morning to proceed on her way. There was a halt of five minutes, and then they pushed on once more, reaching Harsova the next day. There they heard that Mejidia and Czernavoda had fallen, and that no defence could be made. Dr. Stanovitch came to see Dr. Chesney and said the position was very serious. He had lost his staff and had no instructions what to do or where to go.

---

1. Dr. Inglis' report.

It was impossible to cross the Danube at Harsova, as all the barges were crowded with troops. Moreover he had no knowledge of the country or the road, and could only advise Dr. Chesney to follow the stream of the retreat with the hope of finding a pontoon bridge at Isakcea. He also gave them the uncomfortable intelligence that, as far as he knew, there was every possibility of the Bulgars swooping down upon them at any moment, as there were no troops between them and the Bulgars. The trek was resumed, progress being on average, about three miles an hour, never more. Fortunately Dr. Stanovitch's advice proved to be sound for they arrived at Isakcea, found the pontoon bridge, and reached Ismail at 3 p.m. on the 3rd November, after ten days of continuous trekking and camping in the open.

Some of the Transport's experiences in this first retreat are recorded in a report from Mrs. Haverfield;

From Bulbul Mic we moved to Bulbul Mare, and after one night were ordered to Alacap. We did not get away till about 10 p.m., as the ambulances were busy between Bulbul Mare and Mejidia. The road was so crammed with retreating troops and weary animals that it was impossible to get through with the wounded, so when the last ambulance came in we made a start for Alacap. Meanwhile the rain poured down, making it impossible to use the field track I had hoped to take in order to catch up the hospital carts (1st Serb Hospital), that had gone on some hours before. We made for Mejidia, from whence I was told there was a good road—a fallacy, as usual,—and, after sticking in the mud decided to wait till dawn. There was the same old mud track up hill and down dale, over which we pushed and pulled ambulances and lorries the whole day, till we reached Alacap, where we found Dr. Chesney and the 1st Serb Hospital.

Here we finally hoped for food and rest. We were told to get ambulances ready for wounded and to prepare a meal. Before we had time to eat it we were ordered off again. . . . Streams of troops, refugees, wagons, guns and animals of all kinds were trailing along all day, and as darkness fell, all converged on Caromarat. The streets or, rather muddy lanes between the houses soon became one mass of terrified humanity, screaming, crying and cursing, cars and scared animals added to the noise, scenes of terror and despair never to be forgotten. We remained in the mud till 2 a.m., when a start was made. At the corner of four cross-roads I found our lorries and Dr. Inglis. We remained in the mud till 2 a.m. when off we went once more.

Dr. Inglis after seeing her seven off from Saragea to Harsova *en route* to Galatz, spent two days and a night in pursuit of her Serb Lazarette owing to the rapid changes in the orders it received as to its destination. Lack of petrol at length compelled her to make for Harsova, where she as asked by Dr. Costinesco (Head of the Roumanian Medical Services), to take charge of a dressing station on the wharf. There she worked and set up a feeding station, but it was only for a day. Dr. Costinesco came down in the evening and said she must go. They left by boat for Galatz the same night, and not too soon, for the next morning Harsova was shelled by the enemy. The transport went with the 1st Division of the Serb Army, which had withdrawn from action, to Ismail.

In the following letter to the London Committee, Dr. Inglis pays tribute to her unit's work:

> In case this arrives before my report, I should like to say first that the committee may be thoroughly satisfied with the work done and the spirit displayed by almost every member of the unit. They worked magnificently at Mejidia and took the retreat in a very joyous indomitable way. One cannot say they were plucky, because I don't think it ever entered their heads to be afraid. In the middle of a panic, when people were actually running along the road and throwing things off the carts to lighten them, and men with their rifles and bayonets were actually climbing on to our Red Cross carts to save a few minutes, our girls in that particular party were picking up the thrown-away vegetables and things they wanted. The last live days at Mejidia, when we were bombed by aeroplanes every day, they did not even stop their work to go and look.

On 30th December the following communication was received by the London Committee from the Secretary of the Admiralty:

> Madam,—I am commanded by the Lords Commissioners of the Admiralty to acquaint you that a report has been received from an officer of the Royal Navy who visited certain ports of the Danube in October last (1916), which contains the following remarks on the Scottish Women's Hospital at Braila

'A camp of the Scottish Women's Hospital was here (at Braila, 28th October), having retreated from Mejidia, where they were nearly forgotten and left behind.

'He, (General Zaioutchowsky), like everyone else had nothing but praise for the Scottish Women's Hospital, whose motor ambulances were the first thing to be noticed on landing at Braila. They have all lost their kits in the retreat.'—I am Madam, your obedient servant,

J. W. S. Anderson
(For. Secretary).

After the withdrawal of the Serb Division and the hospitals from the Dobrudja, Dr. Inglis was asked by the Russian Red Cross to work with them, which she agreed to do, with the concurrence of the Serbs, who told her that the best work she could do for them was to help the Russians while the Serb Division was resting. The transport was therefore attached to the 3rd Russian Division, and on the 30th of November sent once more into the Dobrudja at Babadagh, halfway between Tulcea on the Danube and the first Russian dressing-station at Cogealak. The cars ran between Cogealak and other villages, picking up the wounded from the clearing stations and field hospitals and taking them to the hospital at Babadagh. Mrs. Haverfield found that the Russian ambulances which were supposed to take the wounded on from Babadagh to Tulcea, either ignored the orders to come in with their ambulances or delayed so long that they could never be relied on for effective help, so she stationed six of her cars at Cogealak and six at Babadagh, and the other between Babadagh and Tulcea. Sometimes the cars would travel the whole distance from Cogealak to Tulcea, about fifty miles.

Miss Onslow (second transport officer) writes:

On one occasion a wounded Russian into the ambulance, and asked the little Russian sister if it really was a motorcar, and would not be satisfied until she got out to look. He knew, poor fellow, that it took two days in a horse ambulance while a motor took only a few hours and saved him much pain.

On the 13th of December the transport was ordered to leave Cogealak and to remove all the patients from the dressing-station and take them to Tulcea. The following account of this experience of the second Dobrudja retreat is given by Miss Onslow:

After two days in Tulcea we were ordered to report at a hospital at Enichioi, a village halfway back to Babadagh. On arrival, no hospital was to be seen or even heard of. So we set off in the dark and mud to find quarters, the best accommodation available being a canteen by the roadside. The next morning we tried to get back to Babadagh, but found it impossible, as the Russian Army was in full and hasty retreat. The road, white, and stretching across the plain as far as the eye could see, appeared to carry an ever-moving ribbon along its surface. On turning back we met a messenger sent to recall us to Tulcea, where the whole transport column was urgently needed to evacuate all the hospitals, there on to barges. We all worked hard, as every patient had to be moved no matter how ill he might be. Some were so bad they died before reaching the wharf. The accommodation on the barge was so pitifully inadequate for the large number of patients who were packed so tightly together that one could not feel sorry for those who died before reaching the barges.

The work done at Tulcea received high praise from the Russian authorities, who sent in a request of it to Dr. Inglis at Galatz. The transport returned a third time into the Dobrudja picking up wounded and evacuating hospitals in isolated parts of the hills, going to and fro under endless difficulties and not without risk of falling into enemy hands, as the Bulgars were in close pursuit.

We evacuated as many as we could take, but in comparison with the total it was a mere handful—men with the dirt and blood still on them as they had come in. My car was crowded with about ten or twelve, piled in anyhow, and how I pitied the rest, limping, weary, crawling despairingly the ten miles to Isakcea.[2]

On the afternoon of Christmas Day the Transport finally arrived at Bulgrad, after three weeks of work and wanderings in the Dobrudja.

---

2. Miss Onslow's report.

CHAPTER 3

Braila, Galatz, and Reni

When Dr. Inglis left Harsova it was on the understanding that she and her staff were to move to Galatz, but owing to the bridge of boats on the Danube being closed they were disembarked at Braila.

Perhaps at no time in the history of the hospitals had there been such a heavy task before the Scottish Women. Braila was one vast dumping-ground for the wounded, who poured in every day; and there were no adequate hospitals. *Cafés* and public buildings were requisitioned, and the wounded made as comfortable as circumstances permitted, but as there were only seven trained doctors in the town before Dr. Inglis' arrival, and already some 11,000 wounded, it was an almost hopeless task. As one of the orderlies wrote in her diary:

> Here an endless flow of wounded. We have put some of the beds together and the men three in two beds, but even then had not enough room. You see groups of hungry, weary men crowding the pavement before every hospital.

Dr. Inglis' report shows that the work was also complicated by other difficulties.

> We arrived here on 25th October We went straight into the hospital the evening we arrived, and helped at the dressings. The next morning we were asked to take over another hospital. Seeing the great need, I instantly agreed. The work has been quite satisfactory, and everybody—doctors, sisters, and orderlies—has worked splendidly. Besides the work in the big hospital we had a house on the opposite side of the road for slight cases where there were no operations—only dressings and we had charge there.

The authorities gave us a very comfortable house, just round the corner, with electric light; and those of us who could not find room here slept in the British Consulate, which is empty.

The work went on at Braila until the beginning of December, and the Hospital Staff were working at high pressure throughout their stay there. On December the 3rd came the news of a move:

To form a large dressing-station near the front. . . . Some French sisters are taking our places here. . . . When I went to say good-bye to the patients they all touched their foreheads with the back of my hand and then kissed my hand. Several of them assembled on the stairs and gave three cheers for England and the Scottish sisters.

Some of the extracts from letters and reports show that the staff of the Scottish Women were watched with great interest, while their capacity for work called forth "everyone's admiration."

An anti-feminist Russian officer who inspected the hospital said:

Now at last I see that women can work.

More qualified was the praise given by some of the patients:

The Russian sisters[3] are pretty, but they are not good; the Eng-lish sisters are good, but they are not pretty.

Their clothes, too, were a source of interest. Dr. Inglis comments on the impression made by their workmanlike rubber boots which were found so useful in the winter mud

We have made friends with many Roumanian women, both in our own hospitals and others. One of them said what they loved about us was our 'simplicity.' We wondered what 'simplic-ity' could mean, and Dr. Corbett suggested it must be our *boots!* There is no doubt our boots have made a great impression. We hear of them on all sides!

The attempt to form a dressing-station "nearer the front" resulted in a further week's wanderings.

Eventually the party reached Galatz in safety and took up work there.

Dr. Inglis wrote:

---

3. The term 'sister' is applied to all women in Russia.

So ended my third and I sincerely hope my last retreat. We thought we should have to go right back into Russia, but orders arrived this morning, to our great joy, to say we are to stay here. The consul says it is the worst news he has had yet, for I am such a bird of ill-omen that he knows that the moment the equipment is unpacked and the hospital arranged the whole town will be evacuated! But I tell him things always go in threes, and that therefore retreats are done with.

We were given a building—a school near the port,—which was in many ways satisfactory, as most of the wounded were being brought up by a barge. The building itself made quite a good hospital for 100 beds, leaving room for a good receiving-room and bathroom, a room for dressings, and an operating-room. The rooms were quite nice and wonderfully clean, and it proved a most satisfactory and necessary arrangement having the mess-room in the hospital, as we were able to get meals whenever we were free.

The wounded were pouring through Galatz at the rate of about one thousand a day, and we got practically nothing but bad cases at our hospital. Dr. Potter has a story that she gave orders for any cases that could walk to come down to the dressing-room, and a few minutes afterwards the door was burst open and a man crawled in on all-fours; that was the nearest we could get to a walking case!

The night we opened we got 100 cases. We bathed and dressed them all and began operating the next afternoon at one o'clock, and then went on without a break until five o clock the following morning. We owe a great debt of gratitude to Mr. Scott. Surgeon to the British Armoured Car Corps, who met one of the girls and asked whether he could be of any use. I sent back a message at once that we should be most grateful, and he worked with us without a break until we evacuated He is a first-class surgeon, and it was a great thing to have him there. The cases stayed in a very short time and we evacuated again down to the barges going to Reni, the hospital filling up, and more than filling up, each time. We had eventually to lay down one room entirely with straw, where we simply put the men in their uniforms after dressing them, and the more serious cases we gradually moved from there to mattresses.

Commander Gregory of the British Armoured Car Corps sent

down a message to us that 'in the last resort he would see us out'; so we were able to work on with quiet minds. M. Ile-achenko, our chief (*Chef de la Croix Rouge Russe avec l'Armée sur le Danube*), left me with a written order to stay in Galatz to the 'last moment,' and then to go to Foltesti.

On Thursday. 4th January, the evacuation officer ordered us to evacuate the hospital I told him our orders were to stay until the 'last moment,' and he said that the 'last moment' had come. He arranged to send ambulances for the patients at eight o'clock the next morning, and we went up to the station to arrange for wagons to take us to Foltesti. We found, however that the line to Foltesti was absolutely blocked, and we could neither get there direct nor by going round by Jassi, for the line was blocked northwards. M Ileachenko had gone to inspect a hospital along the Jassi line, and no one in the office could give me any instructions While I was there, debating what to do, Commander Gregory sent down a message to say that he would take us all over to Reni in a barge which had been given him for his corps. We therefore cleared out all the equipment on Thursday afternoon, and the personnel went that night, except four who stayed to evacuate the hospital the following morning.

The committee will not be surprised to hear that at least half the staff came and asked for leave to stay; in fact, one said she thought the whole twenty-two ought to stay. Late that evening, when I went down to the barge to see how the loading was getting on, Mr. Scott came up with a fresh message from Commander Gregory that he did not wish any of us to stay. However, it was obviously impossible to leave the hospital, which at that moment contained sixty-six cases—every one of them bad cases—and I assured Mr. Scott that we would find our way out. As a matter of fact, this was not necessary, for another barge belonging to the Armoured Car Corps went next day and we came off in it.

I have so often said to the committee that the unit works splendidly, that I am afraid they will be rather tired of the phrase. But I cannot possibly allow the work which was done at Galatz to pass without special mention of the magnificent way in which everybody worked. Nobody was off duty; the night nurses staved on until they went to bed, and the day nurses stayed on for most of each night. Most of us got only two or three hours' sleep each night. Dr. Scott pointed out to me that we operated thirty-six hours on end the first day, with three hours' break in the early hours of the morning—and as we had been working twenty-four hours before that admitting, bathing, and dressing—you can imagine what a time we had. Dr. Corbett has also been calculating, and she says we worked sixty-five hours on end with two breaks of three hours' sleep! We came out of it very fit—thanks to the kitchen staff who had food constantly ready from early morning till late at night.

Reni, which was to be the home of Hospital "A" for the next eight months, proved a dreary and cold spot during the winter. The matron wrote:

This is on the banks of the Danube, windswept stretches of bare, undulating ground, a station and barge port. On the north, half a mile away, a queer old-world town, and to the south railway lines, where there is nothing but barracks.

One of the unit described the new quarters in a letter:

Our hospital is a one-storied building, light and airy, built of wood. We are living in a pagoda-like house, quite nice, and we have the most lovely views across the Danube, and to the hills beyond. The guns were very loud and near during the fine weather, but we have not heard them since the cold weather began.

Though the staff quarters were only a short distance from the hospital the severe weather sometimes made the journey between the two buildings one of considerable difficulty. Dr. Inglis wrote:

One snowstorm nearly cut the house off from the hospital owing to the great drifts between. I wish we could have got you a photograph of the staff struggling over to roll call in the morning in their top boots, short skirts, and peaked *barliks* (hooded capes) over their heads. The Danube has been frozen over, and the carts for the wood crossed over on the ice. That is another photograph I wish I could have got: streams of men carrying wood across the river. They say that it has not been frozen for seven years.

The freezing of the Danube was, however, considered a happy circumstance by many of the staff. Owing to the inadequacy of the well, they had hitherto used Danube water for culinary purposes. One of the sisters wrote:

> We have our tea made with boiled snow now; it is much cleaner than Danube water, and tastes nicer.

And an extract from an orderly's diary is even more explicit:

> It (*i.e.* the Danube water) is the same colour as tea, only it is opaque instead of clear, and by now we know our Danube too well to enjoy drinking it. Soup made with it looks lovely, so nice and thick.

Dr. Inglis felt that the hospital was fulfilling its purpose, as a quotation from one of the reports shows:

> The work we are doing is to take in the badly wounded men from the Evacuation Hospital. (All the rest are sent on in ambulance trains.) It is work we are especially fitted for, with our well-equipped theatre and our highly trained nurses, and the committee may, I think, feel satisfied that that hospital is in a very useful niche for the moment.

But in spite of this, she was anxiously awaiting an opportunity to rejoin the Serbs, for whom she had originally been sent out. Early in February, therefore, she went up to Odessa to see what the future of her own division was to be. But the visit proved clearly that at present the Serbs did not need her hospital. They impressed on Dr. Inglis the fact that she could best help them for the moment by helping the Russians, and she therefore returned to Reni and carried on the work there, an "Act" having been signed by the Russians that they would at once release the staff whenever the Serbs required their services.

Under this arrangement, Dr. Inglis was still working in Reni when the Russian revolution broke out in March. The spirit of unrest and indiscipline, which manifested itself among the troops, spread also to the hospitals, and a Russian doctor reported that in the other hospitals the patients had their own committee, which fixed the hours for meals and doctors' visits and made hospital discipline impossible. But there was no sign of this under Dr. Inglis' kindly but firm rules. Without relaxing disciplinary measures, she did all in her power to keep the patients happy and contented and as the Russian Easter drew near, she bought four *ikons* to be put up in the wards, that the men might feel more at home. The result of this kindly thought was a charming Easter letter written by the patients to the—

Much-honoured Elsie Maud, the daughter of John. The wounded and sick soldiers from all parts of the army and fleet of great free Russia, who are now for healing in the hospital which you command, penetrated with a feeling of sincere respect. feel it their much desired duty, today, on the day of the feast of Holy Easter, to express to you our deep reverence to you the doctor warmly loved by all, and also to your honoured personnel of women. We wish also to express our sincere gratitude for all the care and attention bestowed on us, and we bow low before the tireless and wonderful work of yourself and your personnel, which we see every day directed towards the good of the soldiers allied to your country. . . . May England live.

(Sgd.)   The Russian Citizen Soldiers.

In consequence of the revolution there was a constant changing of troops in the neighbourhood and it was this, combined with the "spy-fever" which had broken out all along the front, that led to a highly disagreeable incident. The curious form in which the staff quarters were built made the building a centre of interest to a newly arrived regiment, and someone spread the report that signalling was taking place from the turret-window of the dispenser's room. Miss Murphy was therefore arrested as a spy, and as Dr. Inglis insisted on accompanying her—since no affirmations of the girl's innocence availed—they both spent the night as prisoners. Much to their indignation, they were not set free until the unit had signed a paper, "guaranteeing the fidelity" of Miss Murphy. Dr. Inglis had meanwhile managed to get word of the arrest through to General Kronpensky, the Red Cross Commissioner, who came up at once from Galatz to put matters right. General Zourikoff, general in command of the army to which the regiment belonged, wired at once:

Please accept and convey to Sister Murphy the expression of my heartiest regret at her arrest, she being one of a unit of the best workers of the British nation.—

Zourikoff.

Dr. Inglis' reply showed that she was determined that the incident should be forgotten.

I desire to express in my own name, in Sister Murphy's, and in that of the Sisters of the Scottish Women's Hospital our heart-felt thanks for your telegram, and for the kind thought that prompted it. It will always be a proud memory to us that we were able to work with the great Russian nation in that war in which our two countries are allied.

After the excitement of the spy incident had died away, time went by uneventfully, and since there was little active fighting there was also a lull in the work. In fact, nothing of interest was reported during the early summer except the reception of two patients from the British Armoured Car Section, which gave the Scottish Women the joy of nursing their own countrymen.

While Hospital "A" was stationed at Reni, the second detachment of the London Units. Hospital "B" had also filled a great need on the Roumanian front. It had left Odessa in March and was attached to the Russian Division at Tecuci, a small town in Roumania about ten miles behind the line. They were given a field to camp in, and a house, which had been used as a Russian and Roumanian hospital, and was indescribably dirty. They set to work and whitewashed and cleaned it, chiefly with their own hands. The hospital consisted of four wards, with ten beds in each ward, a theatre, dispensary, and dressing-room. They had surgical cases, mainly bombing accidents from aeroplanes, as there were constant raids from enemy aircraft.

The first week in July, Hospital "B" moved forward, right up to the front to Varnitza, a small hamlet in a valley of the Carpathians. Here they were told by the Russians that there was to be a great advance, and Dr. Chesney put up hospital tents for the patients, and for the staff, consisting of two doctors, two sisters, x-ray assistant, matron, an interpreter, and three orderlies.

A member of the staff wrote:

We were surrounded by Russian big guns. The enemy being entrenched on a slope of the Carpathians commanding our valley, we were told that the valley would be shelled and that we must make dugouts. This it was quite impossible to do, as we had neither enough time nor men. The noise of the guns was deafening. Soon after our arrival the Russians succeeded in driving the enemy out of their position and forced them back some distance. After remaining there ten days we were moved forward again to another valley, where we camped for about a fortnight. The Germans shelled our valley every day, but we were safe enough as long as we kept under the shelter of the hill—the shells used to burst in the river bed. At length it became obvious that the Russians would not fight, and as the shelling became more violent the Russian general said we must go.

We had to travel by night, the roads being shelled by day, until we reached Tecuci; there we rested for a couple of days and resumed our journey by night to Reni, where we joined Dr. Inglis.

As the summer progressed it became evident that the whole unit would shortly be rejoining the Serbs; but this was not to happen without one further rush of work, brought about by Kerensky's gallant effort to promote a sustained offensive all along the Russo-Roumanian front. For a few weeks there was heavy fighting, and Reni was once more a great hospital centre. When the rush took place, Dr. Inglis was absent in Odessa negotiating with the authorities about rejoining the Serbs; but Dr. Laird took charge and organised the hospital to meet the greatly increased number of patients so well that the work suffered little by the absence of the chief.

Despite the revolution the hospital had managed to work smoothly, and, except for the one untoward incident, relations with the Russians both before and after the great upheaval had been friendly and sympathetic. Everyone appreciated the work done, and much regret was expressed at the departure of the "English Sisters" from Reni.

CHAPTER 4

Back With the Serb Division

The letters and reports received from Dr. Inglis during the last months of the unit's work in Russia, though necessarily brief and guarded in their expression, reflected the anxiety she felt with regard to their future work with the Serbs.

The chaotic condition of affairs in Russia, and the disorganisation of the Russian Army consequent on the revolution, had convinced the Serb Command that if fighting were renewed there could be no hope of an effective stand being made by the Russians, and the only result of the Serbs going into action would be to expose themselves to another disaster such as they had experienced in the Dobrudja.

"The men want to fight," said General Zivcovitch to Dr. Inglis; "they are not cowards, but it goes to my heart to send them like this to their death."

Dr. Inglis had had ample evidence herself of the demoralised condition of the Russian soldiers, and had ever reason for fearing that the Serbs would be sacrificed uselessly. She wrote:

> They are such a fine body of men, and are anxious to go to some other front to fight where they can rely on support.

Early in July there seemed every possibility of their being allowed to leave Russia for Salonika, but on the 26th the Russian Headquarters definitely stated that they needed the Serbs on the Roumanian front. On hearing this, Dr. Inglis instantly sought the intervention of the British authorities at home for obtaining permission from the Russian Government to have the Serbs transferred to another front. The Serb Staff was powerless in the matter and entirely dependent on the good

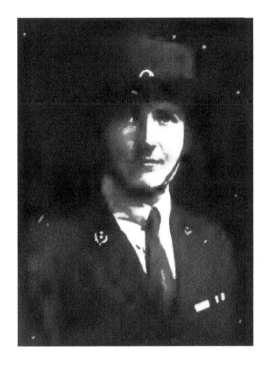

Miss E. Frances Robinson

offices of the British Government for effecting their release.

Dr. Inglis wrote in July, from Odessa:

> I am up here to see what I can do to get this miserable tangle undone. They want the division to go to the front 'to encourage the Russians.'

Unfortunately, many more efforts had to be made by Dr. Inglis before the "tangle" was finally undone. The negotiations between the Russian, Serb, and Roumanian Commands (the latter being more unwilling even than the Russians to let the Serbs go) went dragging on for months—months of anxiety and uncertainty, aggravated by continual disappointment, as the orders to leave Russia would often be contradicted the next day.

It was at this juncture that Dr. Inglis conceived the plan of conveying to the home authorities some account of the real state of affairs, and at her suggestion Dr. Jambrishak (Member of the Jugo-Slav Committee), then in Odessa, drew up a report of the political situation as it affected the Serbs. This report was given to Miss Robinson and Miss Holme, members of the transport, who were returning to England.

To carry away any written document, especially of such a confidential nature, was, however, impossible, so Miss Robinson committed it all, some 2500 words, to memory. On a small piece of paper about an inch square the headings of the report were written out and secreted by Miss Holme in a needle-case. In this manner a detailed account of the position of the Serbs was conveyed from Russia.

Dr. Inglis also sent a message to the Foreign Office through Sir George Buchanan, British Ambassador at Petrograd, to the following effect:

> Dr. Inglis informed the Foreign Office that orders had been received from the 1st Serbian Division not to proceed to Archangel, but to go to the Roumanian front. This change was made at the urgent request of the Russian general, the reason given being that the Russian troops required stiffening by the Serbians Dr Inglis expressed the opinion that it would be sacrificing the Serbian Division to send them into action, as the Russians were completely disorganised. Most of the wounded Russians in her hospital had self-inflicted wounds in the left hand. It would require several army corps to stiffen the Russians. The present condition of the Serbians was deplorable, and in the coming winter the question of supplying them with food and fuel

250

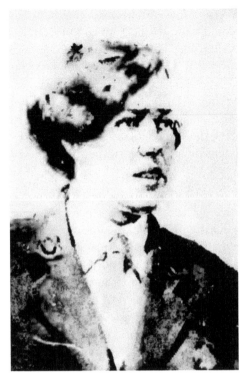

MISS VERA HOLME

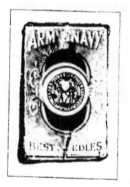

SCRAP OF PAPER AND THE NEEDLE-CASE

would be a very serious one. In any event, the Scottish Women's Hospitals would stand by the Serbian Division, and would accompany them if they went to the Roumanian front."

Lord Robert Cecil. Under-Secretary for Foreign Affairs, replied through Sir George Buchanan that he would do what he could to carry out the wishes of Dr Inglis, but the final decision must rest with the War Office.

At the end of the month of August the unit rejoined the Serb Division at Hadji-Abdul, a little village midway between Reni and Bulgrad.

Dr. Inglis described it as:

A lovely place . . . and we have a perfectly lovely camping-ground among the trees. The division is hidden away wonderfully under the trees, and at first they were very loath to let us pitch our big tents, that could not be so thoroughly hidden, but I was quite bent on letting them see what a nice hospital you had sent out, so I managed to get it pitched, and they are so pleased with us. They bring everybody—Russian generals, Roumanian military *attachés* and ministers—to see it, and they are quite content because our painted canvas looks like the roofs of ordinary houses.

Although there were no wounded, there was a considerable number of sick, chiefly malaria cases, which kept the staff fairly busy.

There was a constant rumour of a "grand offensive" to be undertaken on the Roumanian front, which Dr. Inglis, though extremely sceptical of any offensive on a large scale, made every preparation to meet.

In a letter to Miss Onslow, her transport officer at Odessa, she asked for the cars, which had been carrying wounded from the station at Odessa to the hospitals in the town, to be sent up to join the hospital at Hadji-Abdul.

No one really knows what the Russian Government means or will do. I don't think the last explanation of how the last order for Archangel came to be altered improves things at all. It shows there is no settled policy, but that they are swayed by the last opinion. Such a wave may carry us right into Roumania, and I want *this* hospital at any rate to be ready, and then one often gets a chance of helping one would otherwise lose. It is awfully rice being back with the Serbs. We had lunch at the headquarters today—six of us—a kind of official welcome.

The London Committee had cabled to Dr. Inglis in the same month advising the withdrawal of the unit, but leaving the decision in her hands, to which she replied:

> I am grateful to you for leaving decision in my hands. I will come with the division.

Following upon this cable came a letter, in which she emphasised her reasons for remaining:

> If there were a disaster we should none of us ever forgive ourselves if we had left. We *must* stand by. If you want us home, get *them* out.

In almost identical words Florence Nightingale answered those who urged her return from the Crimea—she would only return when the last of her wounded could be moved with her.

On September the 28th news was brought to Dr Inglis that the division was to leave in three days for Archangel. The few days extended to a month, for a counter-order came for the division to proceed to Ackerman. near Odessa, on the Black Sea, there to remain until the spring.

Matters had now become rather serious for the unit. Dr. Inglis had shown signs of failing health, and there was not much hope of obtaining adequate supplies of the bare necessities of life, food, fuel, and clothing for the coming winter. With characteristic courage Dr. Inglis and her unit faced the situation. A member of the unit describes an interview she had with Dr. Inglis on the day when the orders came for Ackerman.

> She told me it was the first time in her life she had ever been homesick. She had written to her people saying it was her last letter from Russia, and now we were not going after all. She then proceeded to tell me how she would arrange the hospital, and who would be sent home and who would remain. . . . Ill as she was, the details were arranged in her mind, and we had only heard the change of plan that morning. . . . I was very miserable when I left her. She was obviously unfit to remain on.[1]

The cold was very great, and an effort was made to find rooms in

1. *Some Months in Bessarabia with the Scottish Women's Hospitals,*—*Blackwood's Maga-zine*, May, 1918.

the village. The unit were most anxious for Dr. Inglis, who felt the cold intensely, to move into a house, but she resolutely declined to do so unless all the members of the unit could find similar accommodation. Fortunately, while the search was being made for rooms an order, which proved to be final, came in that the division was to leave for Archangel.

The British Consul at Odessa had been asked by Dr. Inglis to send a message to the Foreign Office to the following effect: That she was on her way home with the Serb Division to Archangel, and that the Serbian Chief of Staff had made an earnest request that if it were possible they might be allowed to pass through England, in order to judge for themselves of the work being done there for the success of the Allied cause. These men, after witnessing the terrible chaos in Russia—a country they had regarded as their protector—were difficult to persuade that conditions were better in other countries. This proposal of sending the Serbs through England was very warmly supported by the Serbian Consul General at Odessa, and was adopted.

Dr. Inglis in her letters and reports often referred to the valuable servicers kindly rendered to the unit by the British Consul at Odessa, who from the day of her arrival was always ready to help in any difficulty. In his letter of farewell to Dr. Inglis he expressed his good wishes for the continued success of the Scottish Women's Hospitals, and added:

Both my staff and myself are very sorry to think you are leaving. The sorrow, though, is purely selfish,—anything that we have been able to do for you or the hospital has been a real pleasure to us. Although we have seen one or more of you on business every day during the past year, never once have the questions asked been anything but practical, nor has assistance been thoughtlessly or uselessly required. Allow me to offer you and your hospital, on behalf of my staff and myself, our best wishes for further successes such as you have so deservedly won on this front. I am sure that any difficulties you have met with at any time are more than compensated by the high praise spoken by all Russian who have come in contact with your hospital.

The London Units Committee had feared greatly for the fate of the unit if, as seemed probable, the Serb Division was not able to leave Russia, and on the 9th of November approached the Hon. H. Nicholson at the War Department of the Foreign Office, who assured them that the unit would be quite safe with the Serbs, who were well disciplined and devoted to Dr. Inglis. At that moment he thought it would be most unsafe for the unit to leave the Serbs and try to come home overland.

Mr. Nicholson expressed the opinion that the committee would never persuade Dr. Inglis to leave her Serbs, and added:

> I cannot express to you our admiration here for Dr. Inglis and the work your units have done.

On November the 14th a cable was received by the committee from Dr. Inglis at Archangel announcing her departure:

> On our way home. Everything satisfactory, and all well except me.

This was the first intimation that Dr. Inglis was ill which reached the London Committee.

A member of the unit who was in close attendance on Dr. Inglis during the weeks of her illness at Hadji-Abdul, and on the journey home, said she was quite convinced that any other woman would have died *en route*—the discomforts were so great. But Dr. Inglis had made up her mind she would bring the unit and the Serbs home; therefore she never allowed the idea of dying to come into her mind.

> I shall never forget her on the journey—never a word of complaint of any kind, although her appearance told you everything she would not.

CHAPTER 5

The Elsie Inglis Unit

During the last days of the voyage Dr. Inglis had had been very ill, but the day before the ship anchored in the Tyne she had dressed and gone up on deck to bid goodbye to the Serb Staff, standing; for about half an hour while the members took leave of her. After this effort she was much exhausted, but remained up till the evening.

When the tug came alongside to take her off the ship, she would not allow herself to be carried, but with the aid of two of the ships officers walked from her cabin and even down the gangway to the tug.

It was a sad homecoming for the unit. In spite of their chief's almost miraculous conquest of physical weakness and pain, they were not deceived as to the gravity of her condition. But that intrepid spirit never for one second relinquished command of the failing body she dominated it to the end. The sword had outworn the sheath and death came next day. She died on British soil, and spoke with those she loved, until her passing.

Her last message to the Chairman of the London Units Committee showed how almost to the very end her thoughts were concerned with the future of the Serbs.

Whatever happens, dear Miss Palliser, do beg the committee to make sure that the Serbs have their hospital and transport, for they do need them.

The committee required no persuasion to carry this wish into effect. They immediately began preparation for the reorganising and re-equipping of the unit, which, after inevitable delays, was ready for service in February 1918. It consisted of a personnel of twenty-five, to serve a hundred beds, and a Motor Transport Section attached to the hospital, with twenty-five cars, etc., and a personnel of thirty-two.

There were three doctors, Dr. Annette Benson, C. M. O.; an administrator, Miss Gwynn; and a Chief Transport officer, Miss Geraldine Hedges.

On 19th February the unit, now named "the Elsie Inglis Unit," had the honour of being inspected by the king and queen.

The members of the unit marched to Buckingham Palace from the committee's offices in Victoria Street, and were drawn up in the grounds of the palace facing the terrace.

The officers of the committee were summoned to the presence of the king and queen inside the palace, and were presented to their majesties. Afterwards the doctors were presented, and the king and queen proceeded to inspect the unit.

The queen spoke to several members of the unit who had been in Russia with Dr. Inglis, especially with Dr. Ward, who had attended Dr. Inglis on her journey home and during her last hours. On bidding the unit farewell, the king expressed his admiration of the splendid courage that had been shown, and cordially wished them a safe journey, success in their work, and a happy return.

The Elsie Inglis Unit went out under the protection and patronage of the War Office, and the journey was easy and delightful, though it lacked something of that sense of personal responsibility and spirit of adventure which marked the journey through Russia. On arrival the unit was transported to the chosen site for the camp, about thirty miles from Salonika, between Dragomantsi and Vertekop.

Hills stood all around the place, and the tents for the staff were on a steep hill backed by great gray rocks. This hill was carpeted with asphodel in the spring, and the whole camping-ground bloomed with meadow flowers. Right round the bottom of the camp, where the laundry tents were pitched, a stream ran fed by an underground spring of clear cold water: it was never dry even in the burning summer, and when the rainy season began, it rejoiced all hearts by a sudden flood racing in full spate. The light railway also ran through the bottom of the camp, and this was a very great convenience, especially on the occasion of the first arrival of the equipment, when the cases and poles were flung out on to the camping-ground.

On Monday, the 1st of April, the unit arrived. The work of preparation for patients went on apace, until on Monday, the 29th of April, the hospital was opened, and the unit received their first convoy of sick and wounded.

On the 20th of September the "Elsie Inglis" Hospital was moved by road up to Donii Pojar. Donii Pojar was situated just behind the lines at the beginning of the attack, but was separated by towering hills from the actual front before the arrival of the hospital there. These hills had been taken by the French and the Serbs in the first days of the fighting, partly by help of rope ladders. The "Elsie Inglis" Hospital was the first dressing-station behind the lines. A great many nationalities were represented among the patients: Serbs, French, Italians, Greeks, Turks. Russians, one Englishman, Bulgars, a German, Austrians, Senegalese, and Arabs.

On the 16th of October the greater part of the hospital staff and its equipment wais transported to Skoplje, the *bolnichars,* following a few days later.

At Skoplje the hospital found quarters in a disused school, with a house in the compound for the staff. No delay was allowed the unit for preparing to receive patients, as the influenza epidemic was at its height and within three days of arrival the hospital was full.

> The sisters and nurses worked admirably, and fortunately we have no cases of influenza among the hospital staff. Though we all suffered from the cold (there was little glass in the windows in the building when we arrived) we were extremely well, and our appetites taxed the cook's powers, as for the first fortnight she had nothing but a hole in a mud oven to cook over.

But the work at Skoplje was not of long duration, for orders soon came for another move, this time to Sarajevo, where they met with a cordial reception from both the local authorities and Serb ladies. The building assigned as hospital (in civil life a boys' school) was still in possession of an Austrian doctor and nurses. As soon as these had evacuated the unit proceeded to bring the hospital up to the usual standard of British cleanliness, an operation involving very hard work. At first patients were received from the Timok division then stationed at Sarajevo, but there was no rush of work as there was already a large Serbian military hospital in the town.

Throughout the period of three months, ending in April 1919, that the "Elsie Inglis" Unit was stationed at Sarajevo, the members received lavish hospitality from local ladies. At the farewell party given by Dr. Chesney, it was evident that as an element in the cementing of the entente between England and Bosnia and perhaps, by this means, between Bosnia and Serbia proper, the unit had done good work, possibly of greater importance than the actual medical work which they had hoped to undertake.

CHAPTER 1

Corsica

The story of the Russian Unit with which Dr. Inglis was so closely associated has been told, and now we must return to Serbia and pick up the thread of the history where we left it at the end of Part 2. The following chapters contain an account of the work the S.W.H. did for the Serbs during their exile, till their victorious return once more to the land they loved, and had fought for so indomitably.

Letter from Dr. Curcin to the S.W.H. Committee

London, January 1916.

Dear Madam,—Hearing of your gracious decision to give us another hospital—this time for the Serbian refugees in Corsica—the Headquarters Staff of the Serbian Army has instructed me to place myself at your disposal to facilitate the installation of this hospital by procuring the requisite information concerning the refugees, or by acting as intermediary between your committee and the Serbian and French authorities.

The Headquarters Staff—and in particular the Chief of the Sanitary Section, who are deprived at the moment of the means of expressing to you personally their profound gratitude—have imposed on me the pleasant duty of explaining to your committee the extraordinarily useful work which was accomplished in Serbia by the Scottish Women's Hospitals during this war. They were, after Lady Paget, the first to come and help us during the very sad time of our worst epidemic. From the moment of their arrival they set themselves to work with vigour, never hesitating or stopping before the danger of infection or death. Four of their members fell victims to this deadly foe, but the only consequence of this was to increase the zeal of the committee and of the newly arrived members. Among the latter was Dr. Elsie Inglis, the Chief of the Mission, who never tired of her labours, but was ever on the quest of new and more arduous work. She was an organiser without equal. It was this modest but indefatigable woman who decided the English and Serbian Military Authorities to leave a large portion of the English Missions in Serbia to look after the wounded soldiers and prevent them from despairing and fleeing, broken as they were, before the enemy across the mountainous land of Albania. Dr. Inglis remained[1] there herself with her doctors and nurses, and now she refuses to return until there are no serious cases in the hospital.

If the existence of Serbia is for the moment in jeopardy, there are still ten million Serbians who may continue to suffer under the yoke of the enemy but who cannot disappear. These people will never forget all that has been done for them by the English and Scottish women during this war, and there will not be a single Serbian heart in which—by the side of the admiration they have always felt for the great British nation—there will not be found a more tender feeling—that of gratitude to the women of Great Britain who have helped them in their sorrow.

(Sgd.)   Dr. M. Curcin.

Chief of the Department for Foreign Missions of the Sanitary Section of the Serbian Army Headquarters.

CORSICA

In August of 1915, a party of Scottish Women, under Dr. Mary Blair, was sent to Serbia to reinforce Dr. Alice Hutchison's Unit at Valjevo. They arrived at Salonika just at the time when the line of blocking hospitals in the north was being evacuated, and when the great work for the wounded Serbs was beginning in Krushevatz. It was too late for them to be sent up country to Dr. Hutchison—what was to be done? Were they to return home? Not at all. The dogged Scottish Women refused to entertain such an idea; confident in the belief that the call to work would not be long in reaching them, they waited for it in Salonika. It was not long before their confidence was justified. They will soon be found on board the ship conveying Ser-

---

1. This letter was written in January 1915; Dr. Inglis and her party returned as we have seen in February.

bian refugees to Corsica, where they were to form the nucleus of a new unit. Their work was to take a novel direction in caring for the refugees and in "nursing back to life a portion of the sorely tried Serbian nation." The Scottish Women were thus to add another and an unlooked-for service to those they had already been privileged to render to Serbia—services which are destined to continue long after the cessation of the war. It is the story of this unit which has to be told here.

Dr. Mary Blair, with her sixteen women, landed in Salonika in the third week of October. They were kept waiting for some weeks without work. The general advice was 'Go home—this is no place for you.' With the usual contrariness of human nature these 'Refills' at once said, 'Well, then, we'll stay and wait and see,' which they did, until the beginning of December. They housed themselves in an old Turkish *harem* on a hill near Salonika and waited.

Dr. Blair's report, written on 23rd December, tells what they did during the waiting time, and how the work done then opened the door to further developments in Corsica:

I shall recount all that has happened since my last report on 4th December.

I had told you that it was agreed to remove all the Serbian refugees from Salonika and to found a colony for them elsewhere. It was decided that we should be the hospital unit for the colony. The first place suggested was Guevgueli, and it was, of course, on Serbian soil. When that site was evacuated another site had to be chosen, and for some time the choice seemed to lie between Volo, on the east coast of Greece, and a Greek island. Volo seemed almost a settled thing, when circumstances changed it all again.

On 9th December Dr. Anderson and I went with Sir Edward Boyle and Dr. Douritch for a four days' journey in the direction of Monastir. He was travelling on behalf of the Serbian Relief Fund to arrange for distribution of relief to the refugees at Vodena and Florina. We went to see the condition and numbers of the refugees and to gain definite ideas about their medical needs. I felt that after seeing them in the various towns I should have some idea about the need of a hospital and about the scope of the work, We had a very interesting trip, spending one night at Vodena and two at Florina. At Vodena there were about 150 families of refugees—about 50 of these requiring immediate help, and the others help in a few weeks.

At Florina we saw the more pathetic sight of the Serbian soldiers who had straggled in over the pass from the region of Lake Ochrida. We found a number of these sitting or lying by the roadside exhausted, hungry, and footsore. Several looked very ill. We bought loaves of bread and distributed them, and to those who were too ill to eat, we gave hot coffee. We also got them new socks and dressed the frostbitten feet of one or two men. Sir Edward Boyle arranged for these men and the six or seven hundred refugee families to remain there till they could be received in Florina. A doctor and two nurses of another unit were sent up to work temporarily—till the refugees were removed. We saw one family, consisting of a woman, a girl, a little boy about three, and a baby about eleven months old. All these had been wounded by the Bulgars by being prodded with bayonets.

While at Florina, Sir Edward told me that on our return to Salonika, our most urgent work would be to get the refugees quickly and safely away. He relied on our unit for that work.

"While we were away Miss Hunter organised the refugee work at the station. I had asked Sir Edward before leaving if he would like us to do it, and would grant us money from the S.R. funds for the purpose. We offered to supply the labour while waiting for our own scheme. On our return from Florina we found everything in working order—a tea and bread stall to feed the refugees on arrival, a tent pitched to house them for the night, and arrangements made daily for motor transport to convey the refugees and their baggage the next day to an encampment put up for them on the land surrounding the Russian hospital. Sir Edward was most pleased with the rapidity with which the work had been organised and carried out, especially amid all the difficulties of getting things done that there are in Salonika. He spent the whole of the next night at the station and acquired a very favourable impression of the party of Scottish Women you entrusted to my care.

Shortly after this, he sent for me, and definitely laid his plans before me An offer had been received from the French Government to give free transport to the refugees to Ajaccio, and to house them there The first lot were to leave almost at once. He asked me to take my party there—a certain number going in each transport to take care of the refugees on the journey. He wished me to be in charge of the medical affairs of the colony. There was no time to cable home for express permission to go to Ajaccio, but that I believed might be assumed, as we had permission to establish a hospital for civilians, and these are the only Serbian civilians that can be helped at present. We sent off the wire to you, and hoped it would be in time to stop the equipment from starting for Salonika.

I saw Sir Edward on Friday last, had to be ready to sail on Sunday, and actually sailed on Monday at three o'clock. So there has been a great rush. The next party will probably be under Miss Culbard, the third with Miss Hunter, and the last with Dr. Anderson, who remains in Salonika.

All of us were busy helping at the Refugee Camp, and there is so much help needed there and at the station that it was not possible to transfer everyone at once. All the Florina families have to be got down this week and passed on to transports as speedily as possible. There are no helpers to do the work except those who, like ourselves, happen to be on the spot.

I was anxious to get the equipment from the Serbian sheds at Salonika, away with us in this ship. I was told it was not possible, but I thought I would try, as it is so likely never to come at all if left behind. I went out to see the *Amazone* the evening after she left to lie off in the bay, and found her holds empty. I asked the captain if he would take the equipment, and he said he would if it were on board at 9 a.m. It was then 6 p.m. I went back to Mr. Behrens, who thought it would be excellent to do so, but not possible. He agreed that I might try, so I went to the British authorities, who were very nice, but could not help at such short notice. They advised me to try the French. Mr. Behrens went with me. The first officials were charming, and promised a lighter at 8 a.m.

They took us to another office where two carts and eight men were arranged for 7 a.m. I went down about seven with Bell and an orderly and found Mr. Behrens, but no carts or men. The carts came about eight and the men never. We found some odd men and got on with the cartage, but mules are not the best beasts when you are in a hurry. The lighter did not appear till nine, but in the end forty-seven packages were got away, about forty of them being our goods. The only things to follow are some bales buried under sacks of flour, and the Barenga equipment, which were all taken to the French Unit camp by the French authorities. Anything we have taken that is not for our use will be quite safe in Corsica. I do not think it would if left in Salonika, as Sir E. Boyle, Dr. Douritch, and Mr. Behrens will all be leaving, and they are anxious to get the stables emptied and everything used for the benefit of the Serbians.

I shall telegraph on arrival at Ajaccio. I should like to know what you would like the hospital called, and any other things that you wish to give us special instructions about.

I am taking medical charge of the refugees on board. I am afraid one woman is going to have her first baby on board before we reach Corsica. We hope it will be delayed till we arrive, but, in any case, I think we can care for her quite well.

I think there will be plenty of useful work for us among the Serbians in Corsica. They expect to have five or six thousand there.

If ever any work could claim the name of reconstruction, that done by the S.W.H. in Corsica has a title to it. It has been the rebuilding of a nation broken and dispersed—the nursing back to life and health of dying men and women and children. The committee rejoice in the work done by their Corsican Unit, and the Manchester and District Federation may well be proud of the unit that bears their name. The following description of Corsica is from the pen of a member of committee who knows the island well:

Corsica is a country where you can escape from the twentieth century and find yourself in a simpler and larger age. It is an island of most vivid contrasts; you can pass from Ajaccio, which is as far as externals go—an ordinary French town—to places like Bonifacio, Sartene, and Corte, where you slip back at once into the seventeenth century. An hour's motor journey will take you from a mountainous waste above the tree-line to a land of subtropical vegetation, where the orange and olive tree flourish, and the air is sweet with the scent of mimosa, and where, along the roads, aloes and prickly pears, wicked and sinister, form the barriers of the fields. . . .

Corsica is traversed from north-east to south-west by a chain

264

of mountains only moderate in height as alps go, few of them exceeding 8000 feet. But rising as they do from the sea-level, their situation gives them an appearance of great height. They are beautiful mountains, beautifully grouped, their higher peaks snow-covered for six months of the year.

Between the orange groves of the littoral and the barren peaks come wonderful forests of chestnut and oak and pine. The chestnut woods are chiefly round the little country villages—magnificent trees most of them. Their nuts are very largely used for food, manufactured, and cooked in various ways. Above the chestnuts come the oaks, and most wonderful forests of larch and pine.

Corsica is covered by a kind of heath, a perfect blaze of colour. How can I adequately describe to you this glory? Six plants, you are told, form the basis—singly any one of them has little scent, together they have one unlike anything else—a fragrance beloved of the Corsican, and hungered for by the exile. They say that the Corsican mariner can smell it while yet miles out at sea. . . .

Corsica's history, like our own, has been 'one long brawl.' From early Phoenician to Roman, from Roman to Saracen, from Saracen to Genoese—many have tried their hand at its government. For a period of about nine months it was an appurtenance of the British Crown.

In this beautiful little island we find the 5th Unit of the S.W.H. doing its work of reconstruction.

On the 19th of December the first transport left Salonika with two members of the Serbian Relief Fund and two of the Scottish Women's Hospitals—Dr. Mary Blair and Sister Walker. Each subsequent transport was accompanied by members from both societies.

The S.R.F. took over the work of housing, clothing, and providing occupation for the refugees. The S.W.H. organised all the medical work in connection with the Serbian Colony.

Dr. Blair had, on landing, requisitioned an old convent, which she had transformed into a temporary hospital. In the one ward were typhoid, appendicitis pneumonia, and maternity cases, being treated as well as possible under trying and elementary conditions—no water, no means of heating except Primus stoves, and no sanitary arrangements. All the refugees, whether of peasant extraction, or otherwise, were destitute. Amongst them were prospective mothers, and even before they arrived in Ajaccio, one baby was born on board the first transport in which Dr. Blair was crossing. He was given the name of 'Abda,'[2] to recall the crossing into exile.

Another born on the day of arrival was christened Napoleon, in memory of the renowned celebrity of the island. Since that day seventy-nine babies have been born in the S.W. H.. and only two have died; the others are healthy and strong, and rival English babies both in health and in beauty. As a result of the exposure and privations suffered, either during the march or during their flights to Salonika, the whole colony was in a weakened condition—luckily no serious epidemic arose After much searching a suitable building for a hospital was found.[3]

This was the Villa Miot in Ajaccio—a white-washed two-storied building with green Venetian shutters, looking directly on to the bay. Here was housed for over three years the hospital which has been the centre of the work of the S.W.H. in Corsica. On the upper storey the maternity ward, with its red tiled floor and wide windows looking straight over the gulf, was the pleasantest room in the hospital. The work grew on all hands. Tents were pitched in the garden for the open-air treatment of the phthisical patients, of whom there were many. For some time a fever hospital was in the Lazaret, a most picturesque and historic building about two miles distant from the General Hospital. It is a building on a point jutting out into the gulf, built in the form of a semicircle of small rooms round a central courtyard, with pathways of flags between borders of white roses. The place is particularly suited for an infectious diseases hospital, as it is practically a verandah hospital, forming shelter by night for the patients who were nursed all day in the open air in the sunny courtyard.

The out-patient department extended from the General Hospital, where it was first instituted, to four dispensaries in picturesque villages in the mountains. In each of these villages a room served as a dispensary, and was visited on different days of the week.

Soon after the hospital was opened in the Villa Miot over 3000 recruits and several decimated regiments arrived from Serbia. They had come through Albania, and after wandering for some

---

2. *Abda* was the name of the vessel that took the first refugees to Corsica.
3. The quotations are from the letter of a member of the staff.

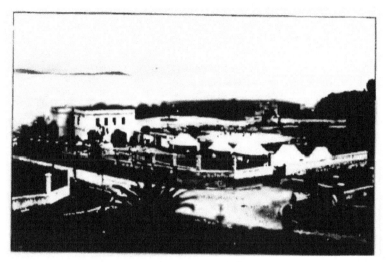

VILLA MIOT, AJACCIO, CORSICA

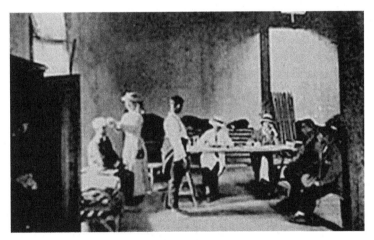

DISPENSARY AT ST. ANTONI

time were finally brought to Corsica. Well do I remember the day they arrived. The *préfet* asked me to accompany him to a review of the men, and welcome them as heroes. But what a pitiful sight they were—broken men; many could not stand up, so worn out were they—some footless, some wounded, all filthy, but game to the last.

These filled up every empty bed in the hospital. Several of us were only too glad to give up our rugs and camp beds to provide more room. The corridors were filled two deep, and the children were placed on the shelves in the linen cupboard to give a few more beds. Two months' rest was granted, and these soldiers, whose ages varied from thirteen to fifty years, were sent on to Corfu to join up with the newly re-formed Serbian Army.

In the same building were German prisoners, who did their best to assist the wounded and stricken soldiers, and to whom we gave medical assistance when necessary.

Our next group of pathetic arrivals was the schoolboys and students who had come through Albania during its time of snow and lack of food. Many of them had had no change of clothes for three months; their ages ranged from six to eighteen years.

Thirty thousand started from Serbia—barely 7000 remained to tell the horrors of the march through the mountains.

From San Giovanni an Italian ship used to put out nightly bearing away to sea the bodies of these boys who during their stay in that town died by hundreds every day. The ship well earned its title *The White Sepulchre*, and the island where these exiles were quarantined came to be known as '*L'Isle des Morts.*'

The work amongst the schoolboys was both interesting and of great value. Dr. Helena Jones was chiefly instrumental in obtaining better conditions for them and she worked hard from early morning until late at night—nothing was too much trouble to her. If you mentioned the boys she put everything aside and flew to their assistance. Many owe their lives, not only to her medical skill, which she devoted to them, but to her breezy way of encouraging and mothering them.

These boys after a rest of three months were divided into two groups, and it was a proud day for the hospital when we cheered 300 fit and strong boys off to school in England, the remainder being sent to study in France.

The story of the Reconstruction Hospital would not be complete without an account of "A Babies' Party" held in its grounds. The writer is Dr. Mary Phillips who was with Dr. Hutchison both in Calais and Valjevo, and was C.M.O. at Corsica when the Baby Show took place.

All the babies who had been born in the Scottish Women's Hospital at Ajaccio were invited to the hospital one afternoon in May 1917.

It was a lovely day, blue sea, blue sky, and not too hot. A tent was pitched in the garden for refreshments and shade. A few friends, including the Serbian Delegate, were invited to meet the mothers and babies, and the committee was represented by Mrs. Gardner Robertson. Amongst the guests were Sir Edward and Lady Boyle. Colonel and Mme. Pitetitch, and Mme. Dedinovatz, the wife of another colonel at the front. Their joy in seeing these vigorous young Serbians was quite touching, and their thanks profuse.

A few mothers and babies came from the hill villages of Uncciani and Boccagnano, but most were resident in Ajaccio, and about forty infants were present. They varied in age, from Napoleon, the first baby born on the island, to the new baby of forty-eight hours (if I remember rightly), shown on my knee in the photograph. The mother was so disappointed that she could not be in the 'slick' herself, and asked me to take her baby, which I did.

The group includes George and Mary, the first babies christened in the hospital, and the famous 'Boozy Bill,' whose name has become a household word among the members of the S.W.H. The *baba* (old woman) in the black head-dress hails from Macedonia, and there are a few in peasant costumes from Northern Serbia.

On arrival, the mothers were received at the front door, passed into the consulting-room, and amid much noise the babies were weighed and weights recorded carefully. It was surprising to find that there was no superstition against weighing such as I often found at home. From the consulting-room the mothers passed into the garden for refreshment and congratulations and much talk over the respective weights of the infants. As far as I remember, they were of average weight; they were naturally fed, for the most part, and all had made good progress.

The previous winter, 1916, had been very cold. The Corsican houses are in it built for cold weather, and many of the children had suffered from bronchopneumonia, but, true to their race, the Serbian babies have wonderful recuperative powers, even after many weeks of fever. We were very proud of the fact that we didn't lose one, and at the time of the party they were all well again.

Little Slobodanka Cistitch was the most wonderful of them all. She was taken ill with pneumonia up at Piana. First Dr. Jackson and then I had to cross the river in spate. The bridge was washed away, and the crossing had to be made in a small boat—after seven attempts, success crowned our efforts. Little Slobodanka was at last brought down to hospital, and after many weary weeks got well and became the pet of the unit.

Now a word about baby clothes. The Serbian custom is to bind the child up 'Italian *Bambino*' fashion, and the straps are most beautifully embroidered, and for peasant babies done in coloured wools. The Jugo-Slavs, of whom we had a fair number, used little hair mattresses and pillows German fashion. In hospital the English method was followed, but I fear that, on leaving, the binding was replaced. One particularly fine baby who had never had her legs bound was proudly shown as the English baby.

In the toddlers' photograph 'Boozy Bill' is marching steadily off to the left with his socks coming down; George in white, in his first trousers, is leaving me, and Mary is on the rig.

Writing of them brings them all back to me, dear little people, with their engaging ways and their caresses for 'Doctor.' How much I hope they are back in their own country. Perhaps you will let me know if the colony has cleared—my godson is there.

The S.W.H. in sunny Corsica brought a whiff of the glen and the heather one day to two exiled Scotsmen, landed there on their way to one of the battle fronts. They saw "Scottish Women's Hospitals" over the gate-posts, and "without a moment's hesitation rushed into the office." A Scotch woman from Aberdeen was in charge that day, and the sense of home that was brought to the two exiles by the Scotch face and the Scotch tongue rejoiced their hearts, though it made one of

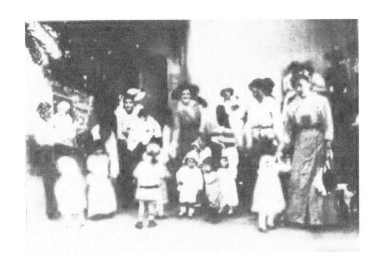

THE BABY SHOW

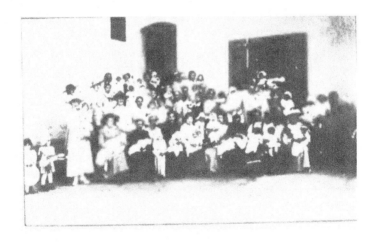

them lay his head down upon the table and cry like a little child.

To many and many a Serb also—man, woman, and child—this hospital has meant *kod kuche*, (home) during their exile.

One boy patient, on being told he was well enough to leave the hospital, begged to be allowed to stay on, saying, "If I leave here, I lose my family again," so much had the place become home to him.

The hospital continued open until April 1919, under Dr. Honoria Keer, who had been appointed C.M.O. in April 1918. The value of the work done will be found faithfully recorded in the lives of many sturdy children in Serbia today, who owe their physical well-being to the love and care bestowed upon their mothers by the Scottish Women in Corsica.

SALLANCHES

At the urgent request of M. Radovanovitch, the Serbian Commissioner-General in France, the committee offered to establish in France a Tuberculosis Hospital for Serbs, which was gratefully accepted. A suitable building was secured at Sallanches, under the shadow of Mont Blanc, and the hospital was opened in March 1918. Marked improvements took place in the health of the patients who were drawn principally from the rank of the Serbian students studying in France, and the number of beds was raised from 100 to 150. Through the generosity of the American Red Cross the funds for the extra beds were provided. Large sums were given by Wales, Greenock, Kilmarnock, and Birmingham, and a ward was called after each of these places.

Dr. Matilda Macphail was the first C.M.O. of the unit, and the Scottish Women owe her a great debt of gratitude for the work she did for them during the six months she was at Sallanches. In the initial stages of the Sanatorium, when many difficulties had to be overcome, her wisdom, commonsense, and organising powers were a great asset to the S.W.H. Dr. Macphail is head of a large women's hospital in Madras, where she spent many years of her life, honoured and loved throughout a wide area. It was while on furlough that she undertook this new duty, giving her time and her ripe experience to the service of the S.W.H., and on her return to India, Dr. Marian Bullock became C.M.O. of the unit. The work continued until May 1919, when the need for this sanatorium was no longer so urgent as it had been.

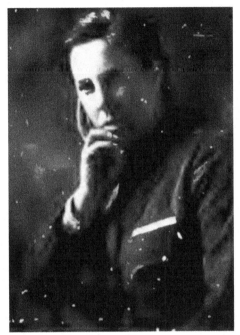

DR. AGNES BENNETT

Ostrovo

THE AMERICAN UNIT

Bruised, battered, and broken, their homes deserted, their country lost, this 2nd Serbian Army was quickly mobilised and thoroughly equipped in Corfu for a crowning effort on behalf of their beloved land.

These words were written of the men of Serbia who had been swept from their country before the advancing enemy, and who were now being gathered together in a supreme attempt to redeem her fortunes The last chapter has told how some of them had filled to overflowing the S.W.H. in Corsica, and had been nursed back to vigour, before they rejoined the army at Corfu for one more desperate venture. The S.W.H were to take part in this venture too, for the Serbian Government approached the Scottish Women's Headquarters with an urgent request for another unit and a Transport Column to accompany the army.

It was to the help of this 2nd Army, fighting in the Monastir district of the Moglena Mountains, west of Salonika, that the Sixth Unit of the S.W.H. was sent in August 1916. Australia was well represented in the unit. The C.M.O., Dr. Agnes Bennett, and two of the other doctors, Doctors Scott and Cooper, Miss Bedford, head of the Transport Column, and several of the orderlies came from that country, and the funds for the upkeep of the unit were subscribed largely in America. It bore the name of the "American Unit." The women of Australia and New Zealand kept the standard of work as high as that set by the medical women in the other Scottish Women's Hospitals.

The unit had a personnel of sixty and was equipped with a view to being as mobile as possible, having sufficient transport, not only for the wounded, but also for the staff. Arriving at Salonika in the middle of August, they were housed for a fortnight at Mikra Bay before being sent up to Ostrovo. It was a busy fortnight in many ways. A canteen was opened at the station in Salonika, which proved invaluable for the short time it was working; some of the nurses were lent to an R.A.M.C. Hospital whose staff had not arrived, and as soon as they could be fitted up, ambulances began to run out to field hospitals carrying wounded and sick. But the most noteworthy piece of work done during this fortnight was the unloading of the equipment in an incredibly short space of time with the result that all was in readiness for the move forward, immediately the order came.

Delay over this particular piece of work would in all probability have prevented that quick move to Ostrovo on 1st September which brought this unit of the S.W.H. to that point on the Serbian Western Front where it was most needed. The story is as follows: The ship bearing the equipment of the unit was to go into harbour at the Greek quay on the Saturday after its arrival at Salonika. There the lorries and Ford vans belonging to the British Motor Transport were to be unloaded, but no provision could be made at that time for discharging the rest of the cargo. The *Fraulein*, as soon as the M.T. cargo was unshipped, was to go out into the bay to await further orders. Rather than allow the equipment on board the *Fraulein* to be carried out into the bay for this indefinite period. Mr. Stebbing,[1] transport officer to the unit, himself determined to unload it, at the same time that the M.T. cargo was being brought on shore.

This was the only chance of securing it, before the uncertain date of the return of the *Fraulein* to harbour. He therefore, with a party of Serbian soldiers and six Scottish Women, started in the morning at 6 a.m., a neck to neck race of uploading their equipment with those who were unloading the M.T. It was an exciting race for the Scottish Women, for whatever of their cargo was still on board, after the last of the M.T. cars was unshipped, would be carried out into the bay, and remain there, until the return of the *Fraulein*. Mr. Stebbing's party worked so well, and the kindly "subalterns in charge of the car-unloading" (after a conversation with Mr. Stebbing) "so arranged matters that as the last car went over the side forward, we slung out the last five slings of tent flooring aft, and the job was done."

---

1. Mr. Stebbing kindly gave his services for the three months that he could be spared from his duties as a lecturer in the Edinburgh University. He did invaluable service for the S.W.H.

The ship had already begun to move slowly as Mr. Stebbing and his kit were hurried down the gangway. That they were justified in their determination to unload their equipment at the first opportunity presented was proved by the fact that the *Fraulein* did not return to the quay until the day *after* the Scottish Women had received orders to proceed to Ostrovo. In Mr. Stebbing's book we read a description of the work the orderlies did in checking the 1400 bales of equipment:

And now I have left the most amazing part of this piece of work till the last, to wit, the performance of the S.W.H. orderlies, for it was magnificent. I have said that a party of orderlies were turned for the nonce into equipment checkers. The whole of the hospital equipment, every box, bale, and piece of tent flooring, was checked by these girls as it came over the ship on to the quay, and rechecked by others as it was stacked up in the dump some fifty yards away. The first party worked from 7 a.m. till 3 p.m., when protesting vigorously that they were not tired and wanted to see the whole thing out, they were relieved and returned to camp.

The second party, four in number, started at 3 p. m. and worked on till 11 a.m. next morning: it is difficult to express admiration for the efficiency of the work they did and the grit they displayed, for they only had about three hours' sleep that night. We did not starve the working parties. The officers of the ship saw to that. It was their unbounded hospitality which made the business a possibility, although they strongly disapproved of the women working in this fashion, and did not forget to let me know it; the girls themselves, however, laughed at them for—well, I think I heard one say 'sentimental idiots.' The mere recital of the way they worked is sufficient in itself. It requires no varnishing. . . .

When you add a glaring hot sun and dense clouds of fine white dust often blown about by a strong breeze, you have a picture of the conditions under which the checker girls worked. They did not appear to consider they were doing anything out of the ordinary. But the French and Italians, officers and men alike, held a different opinion. For they watched them at first with surprise and incredulity. Which changed to admiration. '*Oh, ces Anglais, ils sont si pratique,*' was the oft-repeated exclamation. Whether this allusion referred to the methodical manner in which the girls worked, or to the fact that we brought our women into the show as well as our men, I never determined.[2]

On 1st September the beginning of the Serbian push towards Monastir was rumoured. "The Bulgars were thrown back slightly—the camp buzzed with the news." Colonel Sondermeyer requested Dr. Bennett to take her hospital up to Ostrovo, where they would be near the fighting on that Western Front—the only hospital given this privilege. Ostrovo was eighty-five miles from Salonika. The journey to it was first across fifty miles of the Salonika plain and afterwards up a mountain track of sand or rock. On a Sunday morning, early in September, the advance party started for Ostrovo:

Our pace was to be regulated by that of the lorries, since it was essential that the convoy should keep together. Of the girl chauffeurs with us two were driving the lorries, and as we carried on down the Monastir road through Salonika that early Sunday morning, we made a party which arrested the attention of all and sundry. The S.W.H. were well known in Salonika, but they had never before turned out quite such a convoy as we presented, nor had they ever had the luck to send one up to the front before. The big lorries run by the girls were the chief centre of interest.

Space forbids us to tell, with any degree of fullness, the thrilling story of that march up the mountains. The pass was little suited for motor transport. One of the big lorries had to be left halfway up, at a corner very difficult to negotiate. It was brought on to Ostrovo a few hours later by "a staff-sergeant of the M.T., who opportunely appeared on the scene at the difficult corner and proved a veritable godsend during the next thirty hours." Mr. Stebbing tells in his narrative how the lorry "arrived before dark, driven by that magnificent man the staff-sergeant, who, somewhat ruffled in temper, said he 'was not taking on another job of that description, no, not for no Scottish Women, nor any other women.' I could well believe it. It was a fine feat." The whole party were up by Wednesday and the pitching of the tents began in earnest.

The site of the camp was perfect. Set in a cut among the lower hills, with the high peaks, so soon to be covered with snow, before and behind us, protected from wind on every side, and

---

2. *At the Serbian Front in Macedonia*, by E. P. Stebbing.

surrounded by large trees, with a spring of fresh water beside us, we felt we had reached our ideal camping-ground. But there was much work to do to get our hospital ready. On our first evening in camp, star shells were being sent up over the enemy's lines, and it was known that great preparations were being made for a big advance. Then the first of very heavy guns wakened the unit one night, and by 6.30 a.m.—our breakfast hour—the great advance which ended in the fall of Monastir had begun.[3]

The unit had arrived just in time. The Battle of Gornichevo and the storming of Kaimatchalan both took place in September. There were a few Serbian dressing-stations in the mountains of Moglena, but no hospital except the S.W.H. nearer than Salonika.

The open green space, the river flowing by, and the elm trees on every hand, made a beautiful setting for this hospital under canvas. Mr. Stebbing says of the equipment:

"It may be said here that our equipment was as near perfect as man could desire when unknown conditions are considered."

The women had their work cut out for them, for they were now a casualty clearing-station.

All this meant that there would be plenty of work for our hospital, and the erecting of ward tents proceeded apace. Five wards holding 40 beds each, with their attendant duty tents, were to be erected, and on Tuesday, 19th September, we opened our hospital with 20 patients, the first of whom arrived in the ambulances of the Transport Column. Next day we again admitted 20; on Thursday 37; and this continued till our 200 beds were occupied.

The cases were straight from the battlefield of Kaimatchalan— 'straight' in this country meant that they had field dressings applied, were carried by hand, or on stretchers suspended one on either side of a mule, to a dressing-station about five hours' journey down the mountain. Here they were placed in a *salle de pansements*, the wound iodined, a suitable splint applied, and they were left lying in rows on straw in a *ladnya* (shelter of boughs) till such time as our ambulances could go for them. Many, alas! were beyond human aid, and a sad enclosure of mounds and little wooden crosses is now all that marks the site

---

3. Dr. Bennett's report.

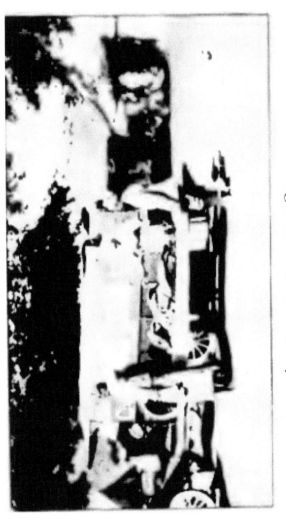

ARRIVAL OF STRETCHER CASES OSTROVO

of the aforetime dressing-station.

The ambulances usually went up and down in convoys, and some nine or ten or fourteen patients often arrived at the same time, hence they had to wait their turn in the Admission Tent lying on their stretchers. We had white 'Reception Tent stretchers,' with white mackintosh over them. This was a special invention of our own, and many medical visitors have complimented me on the system. The patient—always in his dirty, blood-stained, war-stained clothes—was put on these, lifted on to a table about size and height of an operating-table, and on this all his clothes were removed, and he was washed, put into clean pyjamas and then transferred to the ward. This was much better than washing in bed, and also much more thorough. We had always meant to give baths to our patients in this tent but they were far too seriously injured ever to think of baths. Sometimes a dying man had to be carried straight to a ward; some, alas!—nine—were dead on arrival.

This was hardly to be wondered at, when one saw the pass which the ambulances climbed down. The journey took some two hours, and was along the steepest of mountain roads, which zigzagged with sharp hairpin bends down the precipitous slopes. Convoys of food and ammunition often blocked the way, but the amount of consideration given to the ambulances was wonderful. Had the cars been loaded, the ascent would have been impossible, for even when empty the ambulances (fortunately light Ford cars for two cases only) had often to be pushed up. The soldiers used to know the difficult corners for us, and sometimes would wait to give a push at the right moment, and the sister attendants also acquired the knack of jumping out at the right moment and giving a push. The drivers had to wait to cool the engines twice always, sometimes oftener.

Only one mishap occurred on this dangerous road. In trying to pass an ammunition convoy, just when there were only a few inches to spare, the inside wheel knocked against a large stone, threw out the steering, and the car turned over the edge. Most fortunately there were no wounded in the car, and both occupants escaped with a severe shaking and a few bruises. The car was put on the road again at once by a contingent of soldiers, and went on for its load of patients who were eventually safely landed at the hospital.

The cases were of the worst possible variety—mostly 'double,' *i.e.* with two compound fractures—two wounds in different parts. One man was reputed to have thirty-five shot holes in him. With a single compound fracture these cases would, many of them, have been considered worthy of special nurses in our home hospitals. We had three nurses to forty patients.

Gangrene was rife, and the constant amputations were a terrible trial in the operating-tent. This was frantically busy—one splendid little nurse knocked up after the first week, and as we could not possibly spare another, the rest of the work of those terrible few weeks had to be undertaken by one nurse and an orderly. It meant working far into every night, for all the ward dressings had to be sterilised in a single small steriliser. The nurses worked absolutely heroically, and so did the orderlies, and the rapidity with which the latter fell into line was amazing. The suitable ones were soon valuable members of our staff. One brave little orderly joined the long roll of victims of malignant malaria, and now a soldier's cross marks her grave in the sad little Serb cemetery in Salonika.

Our first regular admission was on 19th September, and in the following eight weeks we admitted 523 cases—of these, sixty died. As soon as a case was fit to travel at all we evacuated to a French Evacuation Hospital near Ostrovo station. At this hospital the patients simply rested on stretchers, and were given some food till an ambulance train could be found with room for them. It grieved us sorely, indeed, to know that the wounds we had cleansed and guarded so carefully would often have to remain unattended two days ere the men could reach a base hospital. Later on, when the pressure became less, the sisters used to beg to be sent with a bag of dressings on the day following the patients' evacuation, to see if they were still waiting for a train. The sisters would take boiled water and lotions, and manage everything themselves. The French doctor always allowed them to dress our old patients.

The chest cases were some of the most trying very little could be done for them, we could only make them as comfortable as possible and keep the wounds clean. One remarkable case was that of an officer who was shot right through; the bullet entered at the lower end of the breastbone and emerged between the lower end of the shoulder-blade and the spine He was greatly distressed on admission, but the quiet and comfort of a bed and pillows and careful feeding worked wonders, and he went out quite fit apparently. The men's appreciation of the beds was very great. '*Dobra, Sestra*,' was the most frequent utterance in the wards. The improvement in the first twenty-four hours was wonderful, and it was always sad work to tell them they must move. There was seldom a bed empty even for a night. Each day we informed our D.M.S. how many we could discharge, and as many were sent in as were sent out.

During those weeks our x-ray apparatus[4] was in great demand, and far into every night we were developing plates, for in spite of most careful treatment and erection of the dark tents, the light seemed to get in in the daytime. One hundred and seventy-two plates were taken and developed, and about 250 cases were screened. There was not a great deal of localising done as we found the track of the bullet so patent in most cases that we thought it more practicable to follow these tracks. In the wards all the trained sisters were working hard at dressings; the tidying and cleaning of the wards and giving food to the patients had to be left in the hands of our orderlies and the Serb *bolnichars*. These soon became very deft, and understood from signs what the sisters wanted done.

The size of a Serbian's appetite after many days in the trenches is better imagined than described. They ate what would serve half a dozen of us, and thoroughly enjoyed it. It was wonderful the improvement; in a few days they began to look quite fat. And with their warm, comfortable beds and regular food, in spite of their wounds they were a wonderfully merry lot, and the chorus of '*Dobra dans*,' when one went into the ward and greeted them all, had a very happy ring in it. The dressings were often terrible—compound fractures with horrible septic wounds needing thorough washing every day. It was often necessary to give anaesthetics and do minor operations in the wards—the number done in the operating-tent was 350.

The operating-tent was a great success, the single marquee with double wall answering particularly well, as the light was so good. This was the gift of the 'Ayrshire Farmers.' We made locking cupboards of boxes for our precious store of instruments, all

---

4. Valuable help was rendered to the X-ray department by Captain Riddell, R.A.M.C., from Salonika.

too few, because we were only equipped for 100 surgical beds. Stools and small tables were made of wood from the equipment cases and packages, and we warmed the tent by having two of the small Lucifer stoves underneath the operating-table. We found these also a great success, and very little trouble to manage.[5]

> Macedonia, 15th October 1916.
>
> . . . Since my last letter we have had the ceremony of the consecration of the Hospital performed by the Serbian Church. The Serbs took a great deal of trouble to make the function a very happy one. Colonel Sondermeyer arranged everything, and the crown prince and his staff, and General Vassitch and his staff, were all present. We also asked the British Liaison Officer to come, but he was unable to do so, and Colonel Bearn represented the British Army for us. After the ceremony the prince went round the wards and spoke to many of the patients. He was really charming in every way. He said many nice things about the hospital, and afterwards sent a message saying King Peter would write to me.
>
> After the promenade round the hospital we had lunch in our mess-tent, especially prepared by the Serbian Staff of the hospital. The prince, though very grave in all his ways, relaxed somewhat, and I think enjoyed himself at all events, he said he was coming back to see us again. He fairly frequently passes here in his car The general is in command of the division to which we are attached, and asked me to dinner the same night.
>
> We have, up to now, admitted 356 patients, and the hospital is full. Each day we receive as many as we discharge. . . .

Shortly after the visit of the crown prince to the Ostrovo Hospital, the following letter was received a the S.W.H. Headquarters:

> Serbian Legation, 195 Queen's Gate,
> London, S.W., 12th February 1917.
>
> Dear Miss Mair,—I had recently again news from Salonika what splendid work your hospitals are doing. His Royal Highness the Crown Prince, during his visit to your 'American Unit' in Ostrovo, expressed to everybody his great satisfaction and admiration for the untiring devotion of your members under

---

5. Dr. Bennett's report.

Dr. Bennett. May I take this opportunity to thank you again, and to ask you to convey our thanks to your organising secretary who is working with such splendid result in America, Miss Kathleen Burke, and through her to the whole American public who are so generously and untiringly contributing to enable your hospitals to carry on in helping our brave soldiers where the need is greatest. We shall never forget this help rendered by the great British and American nations to us in the time of our fight for life or death.—Yours sincerely.

Jov. M. Jovanovitch,
Serbian Minister.

The S.W.H. Transport Column, under Mrs. Harley had its camp in the village of Ostrovo, two miles distant from the hospital. It worked along the same roads as the ambulances attached to the Hospital, and did very valuable work now and later. Its story is told in another chapter.

For a description of a dressing-station and of the roads along which the cars had to be driven we are indebted again to Mr. Stebbing. "And these little Serbian dressing-stations themselves—the Great War could show few better illustrations, few more pitiful or pathetic illustrations, of what are to all intents and purposes the front line of the Medical Service, than the dressing-stations of the Serbian Army out Gornichevo way or on the Drina below Kaimatchalan during September 1916.

The Gornichevo dressing-station was the first one to which our ambulances went up. It was moved up as the army advanced, but the name may be left to it. Picture a handful of small bell tents, mostly old and in poor repair, pitched at the side of the mountain road the ground-earth or rock-inside covered with a thin layer of straw; and on this straw lay the wounded, the severely wounded cases, many already beyond the help of man even when armed with the highest surgical skill. There was no room for the sitting cases inside the tents, although many of these had bad wounds. They lay or sat outside on a little straw whenever that could be procured. Hard by was a slightly larger tent the floor of earth or mud, which formed the mess and sleeping accommodation of the Serbian Medical Staff of the station.

There was no luxury here. The Serbians doctors led a hard, se-

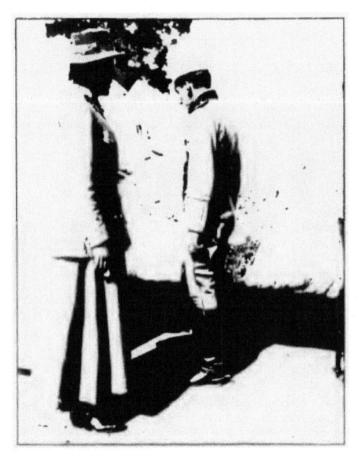

CROWN PRINCE OF SERBIA AT OSTROVO

vere, campaigning life, accompanied by a terrific stress of work as the wounded poured in the tiny station, in, numbers which often entirely swamped its power to deal with them. Up in this place the wounded lay alter receiving dressings, until they could be removed to the Casualty Clearing Stations. From the day of the fight for Gornichevo crest, this station, with the shortest interval of rest, usually utilised in moving forward to keep pace with the advance—the rapid advance—of the fighting Serbs, was overflowing with wounded. The majority of the sitting cases were removed in carts, in fact every sort of conveyance procurable.

Those who could walk were dispatched on foot. The greater number of the severely wounded were removed in the ambulances of Mrs. Harley's Transport Column and our own, and were brought down to our hospital. The number of lives which the hospital saved for the Serbians must have been considerable in those days of severe fighting both from here and from Kaimatchalan. Too high praise cannot be given to the Serbian doctors who had charge of these dressing-stations, for the manner in which they performed these first dressings. They earned high commendation from our own doctors and R.A.M.C officers alike. . . .

The road to Gornichevo was an extraordinary track for an ambulance car, even a Ford one when we first made its acquaintance. And, mind you, all the ambulances were driven by the girl chauffeurs . . . .But the road to Gornichevo, bad as it was, was nothing to the Drina. I have said that this was the dressing-station below Kaimatchalan (where the big fights of 18th to 30th September took place), situated some 5000 feet up the mountain-side. I have seen a great deal of the Himalayas, both eastern and western, and have tramped and ridden miles in these beautiful mountains on tracks and bridle-paths rocky enough, and steep and narrow enough, to please anyone.

But it never entered my head in those days that I should see cars using, and be in cars using, such tracks. I should never have thought it possible that cars would negotiate such tracks. And yet this is what the S.W.H. girl drivers had to do on the Drina, probably the finest feat girls have ever done. . . .That we did not have serious accidents is due as much as anything else to the skilful driving and extraordinary coolness of the girl drivers.

In October some reinforcements were sent from Scotland to the personnel of the Unit. From the diary of an orderly, who afterwards became a driver in the Transport Column, we get some "snapshots" of the life in the camp. She describes her arrival:

Passed right along the very edge of the water for several kilometres and stopped at the station of Ostrovo. White sand on the shore of the lake bright in the moonlight—a row of tall poplars shadowed against the water beyond. Not a soul to be seen on the platform at first; later on a girl with a lantern in a straw hat appeared—R——,of the Harley Unit. Mrs. Harley, General French's sister, had a motor ambulance unit here at Ostrovo, sent out by the S.W.H. She also ran a kind of canteen for feeding the soldiers to and from the front, as they came through in the trains. . . . A short wait of two hours—from 2 till 4 a.m. at R——'s camp fire, at one end of the station—cocoa and gingerbread. Drive to Dr. Bennett's Hospital, about four and a half kilos back along the side of the lake, in a Ford van driven by a girl with short hair and very short skirts, at a furious pace along through the roughest of tracks, with awful bumps and bounces.

Arrived at hospital camp very much shaken up. White tents amongst a clump of great green trees—moonlight—white-capped night sisters with lanterns. Lay down in their tent till the morning. Morning light in the elm trees—magpies—white tents—high mountains beyond. Cocks crowing hoarsely. Guns from behind a big mountain ranger in the north, Kaimatchalan. Interviews with Miss Jack, administrator, and afterwards with Dr. Bennett. On duty in the wards. . .

The hospital ambulances—at that time four were running— and the cars of the Harley Unit at Ostrovo village brought the wounded in from the dressing-stations. One of these was high up on the slopes of the mountain of Kaimatchalan, which had been captured by the Serbs a week or two earlier—the other one at the foot of the mountain. We are about due south of the Moglena Range, of which Kaimatchalan is the highest. . . Our hours on duty are—up at 6 o'clock, breakfast at 6 30, on duty 7.30. Off duty about 7 in the evening. About two hours off during the day. Dancing reels in the mess tent after duty hours, for which I had to supply the music from an old violin costing 30 *francs* bought in Salonika. . . . Moonlight nights. Sad-sounding train whistles in the mountains. Later on an American engine with a siren which wailed wildly through the darkness. After dark, hour-long intoned recitations of national songs coming from the Serb Camp accompanied by the '*guslar.*' . . . The *guslar* is a one-stringed instrument shaped like a *mandolin*, but longer, and held between the knees and played with a bent bow shaped like a double bass bow. . . .

1st November.—Went up to the upper dressing-station as attendant orderly in a car driven by one of the chauffeurs. An awful climb and tremendously rough and narrow tracks up the mountain—boiling engines. A great and wonderful view over the Macedonian Plain towards Mount Olympus, and of the whole lake of Ostrovo. Track up the hill crowded with many coloured throngs of transport of various nations—Serb, French, British, native Turks, and Macedonian. Donkeys, mules, oxen, horses, carts. Ford vans, and our ambulances. The little village of Batechin halfway up, the inhabitants of which are Roumanian. Curiosity of native children about our clothes, especially our stockings. They kept lifting the hems of our skirts to see exactly what we wore on our legs. A great desire to know whether we had any hair on our heads under our caps.

The dressing-station high up on a ridge of the mountains. We brought down two stretcher cases, one of them Milenko, who was put in our ward and became a great favourite. For about a year afterwards he used to send postcards from Bizert in Africa, where he was sent to convalesce. Coming back in the twilight.

19th November.—News of the fall of Monastir. Many nights playing to the Serbs in our wards. Learning Serbian songs. Also sometimes to the British Tommies, invalids from the M.T. companies who were in one of the wards. Sunday services—Dr. Bennett officiating. Playing hymns on the fiddle—there was no other instrument.

January.—I had one of those innocent standing jokes with him (Marko, a patient in the ward) that went on all the time. The idea was, that his heart sometimes departed from his body and went away to visit his wife and children in Serbia, so that when I tried his pulse there was nothing to be felt. But after a minute or so it returned, and then it was my business to tell him the

288

news that it had brought from Serbia—whether his wife and two sons were well, but most important of all, whether or not Mileva had run away with a '*Schvalia*' (German). He always insisted that she had, but that he had remained faithful still; and it was my duty to contradict him and assure him that she was always thinking about him.

Dushan. who lay in the opposite bed, quite a youth and very bright and merry, was always very much pleased with this performance.

On 19th November Monastir fell, and after the splendid advance of the Serbs on Kaimatchalan (8284 feet) the hospital was left behind.

To connect it again with the advancing army an outpost of thirty beds was opened by Dr. Bennett at Dobroveni in the beginning of January 1917. Dr. Cooper was in charge, and volunteers from amongst the staff at Ostrovo were sent in turn to work there. Dr. Bennett reports favourably on this piece of work when writing on 11th February:

> I have good work to report, done by the outpost operating station—so good that the Russians (a number of whom had been admitted) have recognised it by giving Dr. Cooper a decoration. I am so pleased that on the Dobrudja side they are not getting *all* the recognition!

To keep up with the still advancing Serbian Army, this outpost hospital was moved in April several miles farther forward, where they worked till October.

We get an account of the place from Dr. Cooper and one of the orderlies.

Skotchivar, September 1917.

The outpost hospital was stationed at first in Dobraveni in Macedonia, on the left bank of the Czerna River, and was then moved to the opposite bank by the French, who wished the Italians and French to be on one side of the river, and the Serbians and British on the other. The station remained there until the end of April, and then, on account of a very heavy bombing attack, we were moved to Skotchivar, about seven kilometres nearer the front, also close to the river. Miss Bedford was at the new camp, and arranged the pitching of the tents, while I remained behind and saw that everything was sent away, and

289

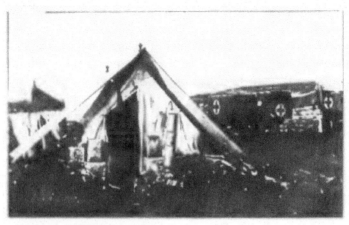

DRESSING STATION AT DOBRAVENI

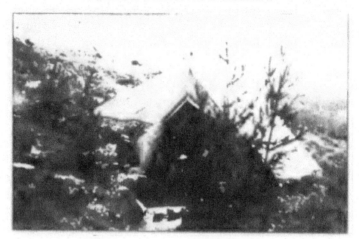

DRESSING STATION AT SKOTCHIVAR

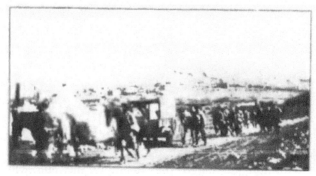

DRESSING STATION AT GORNICHEVO

cleaned up rubbish, and burnt off the incinerator, so that a tidy camp was left. We were not so fortunate at the new site, for it had been a horse camp, and it took us days to clear up old tins, paper, and pieces of clothing.

When the hot weather came on the flies also began, and before long millions were everywhere; all our efforts were very little use. Wire fly traps, issued by the Red Cross, were amongst the most useful methods of destruction. We succeeded in keeping flies out of our storeroom, which was partly dug out and built up with stones, roofed in with wooden beams and a tarpaulin. We lined the whole of this with mosquito nets, and with a few fly papers; there were never more than about a dozen to be seen. We treated the kitchen in the same way, but it didn't avail much, as the door was constantly open and the flies rushed in. There the trouble was, that whatever we did, they got into the food, and it was not an uncommon thing to find an odd fly in your pudding.

The work at this dressing-station was very good for three or four weeks. . . . When I left on 20th August, twenty-three beds were occupied out of thirty-six, and all the patients were in a satisfactory condition. The bomb wounds, in my experience, were the worst; so many of them developed gas gangrene, and were most difficult to do anything with.

The thanks of the whole dressing-station are due to Captain Radivanovitch for his unfailing kindness to everyone.[6]

From an Orderly's Diary

4th June.—Left Ostrovo with three sisters and one other order-ly. A very slow journey by rail, round the lake to Sarovitch and on to Banitza, where we were met by two French cars and con-veyed the rest of the distance to Skotchivar The camp itself was about a kilo on the near side of the village, in a small bare glen. It was on the north slope and caught all the sun from the south. . . . Many of the tents were right on the steep side of the hill . . The dressing-station consisted of thirty beds and an operating theatre. There were some tremendous dust-storms at this time, winds sweeping down the roads so that you couldn't see a yard in front of you. The chauffeurs used to come in with face, hair, eyebrows, and eyelashes thickly powdered with yellow dust.

---

6. Dr. Cooper's report.

On several occasions the tents were blown flat, and letters and papers were swept all over the hillside. One of these hurricanes was accompanied by tremendous sheets of rain, in the midst of which several tents went down. In about ten minutes all the low ground below the camp was in flood and a dashing river was rushing down the little gully beside the kitchen, carrying pots and pans along with it as it went. The rain generally cleared the air a little and killed the flies, but on the other hand it put out my incinerator fire, so that I could not personally welcome it. We all suffered from tremendous thirst at this time, and the only thing for it was to drink gallons of weak tea, as the water, which had to be boiled, was hardly ever cool enough to be pleasant for drinking. . . ."

The hospital at Ostrovo and the dressing-station were not infrequently raided by German aeroplanes; the women at work paid little heed to the bombardments.

> Ostrovo, 24th September 1917.
>
> . . . I wonder if you ever received a letter from me reporting how Dr. de Garis, Sisters Saunders and Angell went on with an operation during an air raid. Sister Saunders continued the anaesthetic, and Sister Angell went on with assistant's work. It was a particularly difficult operation, extracting a bullet from the back of the palate. Only those who know what it is to have bombs falling all round them can realise what an amount of presence of mind and courage such a thing takes. There were fifteen aeroplanes aiming at them, and the camp next to them, which suffered very badly. The girls' presence of mind and courage during air raids and bombardments have been a source of amazement and admiration to me. No one ever wanted to go to the shelters when the whistle used to blow. It was really quite hard work to get them out of the wards. . . .
>
> Agnes Bennett.

In September 1917 Dr. Bennett was obliged to resign on account of ill-health; her place as C.M.O. was taken by Dr. de Garis.

Writing from Cairo on her way to Australia, Dr. Bennett says:

Dear Mrs. Russell,—. . . I am safely thus far on my journey, and am now awaiting a transport to my part of the world. . . . I do hope the unit is getting on well—my heart is still in it. . .

.. I was given an exceedingly nice send-off by the Serbs, who spoke most appreciatively of the hospital. At the dinner at Ostrovo they had a Russian officer who made a speech of thanks (in Russian) for what we had done for his troops. I hope I shall be able to tell you in person some day.   Agnes Bennett.

For another year, until November 1918, the hospital remained at Ostrovo and did good work, principally medical. In November it moved to Vranja in Serbia where under Dr. Emslie it has had a very interesting career. This is given in detail in another chapter.

The quotations which follow are from Dr. de Garis letters, telling of the work during the year November 1917-1918, whilst the unit was still stationed at Ostrovo, and of the violent storm which swept the camp in February. The patient's letter with which this chapter closes is touching. Through the broken English, one feels the ready appreciation of any service rendered, and the genuine gratitude for it so characteristic of the Serb.

Ostrovo, 24th October 1917.

...We are allowed by Colonel Stoitch to admit soldiers of any nationality, and also civilians. I have not done the latter to any extent (save for a run of about six or eight very ill with malaria during Dr. Bennett's illness at the outpost station). However, I have opened a ward of ten beds for women and children, and have admitted two women into it two days ago. These women had previously been treated by us at their homes. Male civilians are put with the soldiers.

Macedonia, 4th June 1918.

... Sisters Angell and Aitken went down on Friday to Salonika, being lent to the Crown Prince's Hospital for a month; at the end of this time I shall replace them with another two. I am going to Salonika tomorrow myself, to attend a medical meeting at which Dr. M'Ilroy is reading a paper, and to see how the two borrowed sisters are faring.

On Sunday we had a number of Serbian children here for the afternoon—we brought them and took them back in our cars—General Vassitch was also present. The children entertained us with Boy Scout drill and some recitations, etc. The patients had made each child a toy—chiefly rag dolls and balls.

The hospital has been very full this week. We have admitted a

293

woman and child today, the first for a long while. I have our full quota of beds up for the military cases (the garage sergeant having devised an ingenious method of mending the beds broken in the storm), and, in addition, have a ridge and pole tent up as an 'extra' for women and children. Without these extra beds, I would not feel justified in admitting civilian cases, owing to the demand for our beds. Our cases are principally medical.

Ostrovo, 26th February 1918.

Dear Miss Kemp,—I cabled to you on Monday about the destruction of tents wrought by Sunday's hurricane, but from my cable you can hardly conceive the condition of affairs here.

To begin with, a week earlier, we had three days' snow, so that the previous Sunday was spent by the personnel in digging their tents out of the snow; then came a thaw and frost, and further thawing, and so on. There is still, indeed, some snow lying about.

Well, on Saturday night it began to rain, and the whole camp was muddy and damp, and tent pegs refused to hold. About 2 a.m. on Sunday began the hurricane; by 3 a.m. most of the unit was up endeavouring to save the tents from collapsing. By 8 a.m. practically every tent in the place had collapsed, the only exceptions being the telephone tent (saved by the devoted exertions of its occupant), the dressing tent, Dr. Rose's and matron's tents, and one tent in Ward V.a, all of which had poles standing and sides collapsed, and Ward I.a (twenty beds), which weathered the storm successfully and was proudly erect. The garage and our kitchen were unroofed, and the patients' kitchen suffered only slightly. The new store (made of flooring and tarpaulin) also came through successfully. The tent stores (groceries, linen, splints, etc.) were scattered abroad. The X-ray and dark-room tents were both in ribbons. Such a scene of desolation has to be seen to be realised.

The unit presented an interesting spectacle also; most of them (including myself) were clad in pyjamas, with stockings drawn over the legs, and shoes and a greatcoat on, and hair streaming wherever the wind listed, but none of us cared!

The patients stuck to their beds till the tents collapsed on them, and even then had to be ordered up. Fortunately no one was hurt, save for a bruise or two.

There were no fires, though we had three narrow escapes. Braziers and stoves were all watered, and great care was taken. Luckily there was no rain, and there was a moon. We counted these three facts our crowning 'marcies.' We have had fine, calm, sunny weather since, also, in which to cope with the situation!

It was obvious that the only thing to do was to evacuate all the patients, and all, except seventeen (convalescent workers or sick *bolnichars*), were dispatched by train. We sent them down in ambulances (no cars were damaged except for their mica windows, some of which were broken), and got them away by the 'Sanitary train.'

Once the patients were gone, we had a 'stand up' breakfast in the kitchen, and then (the storm was now lulling) had Ward V.a fixed, and the fallen part erected, to serve for the convalescent patients, and for a sewing-room for mending tents. Into half I.a we put all bedding and the other half served as a mess-tent. My this time we were really a merry lot, as the storm was over, the patients were gone, and we had been fed, and had nothing but ourselves to worry about. Sister K—— had been transferred from the sick-tent to a Serbian hut, kindly lent us by the interpreter.

I examined all tents cursorily, and all the *bolnichars* having been sent over after lunch by the Serb commandant to be at our disposal, I decided to erect the mess-tent (after mending), the sick-tent, two of the magazine tents, and most of the occupied personnel tents. Of the last all except two had to be put up without their flies, and nearly every tent erected needed some mending first. All the least torn were first dealt with.

At the present moment, *i.e.* in three days, we have the whole of Ward V. up, half of it furnished and full of patients, and the whole of Ward I. up and half of it ready for patients (half is a temporary 'magazine' and sewing-room). The sick-tent and women's ward and half of Ward II. a are also erected, but of these three only the sick-tent is furnished. The theatre and reception tents are ready for use, so we are again a hospital.

I anticipate getting beds ready at the rate of twenty per day, until we have 120; after that the difficulty will begin, as two ward tents (*i.e.* 20 beds) are so badly torn that I scrapped them and used their canvas to repair others, and two more are very unlikely to repair, and will certainly take a long time to get into order.

The X-ray and dark-room tents at present appear almost hopeless, but we *may* get one makeshift tent out of the two.

Of course our great fear is another hurricane though we can hardly have such bad luck again as to strike another thaw at the same time. Our newer tents collapsed as well as our old ones, but they did not tear as the old ones did.

Of course the electric installation is, at least temporarily ruined, but the engine is all right, so some weeks should again find it working.

The dispensary suffered rather severely, bottles being broken, and their contents hopelessly mixed

In the store some homemade jam was spilled (a loss a jamless unit deeply deplores) and scores of eggs were broken. We had just got a big supply the day before the cyclone. All thermometers and glass syringes and medicine glasses were broken, with an occasional exception.

I am sure we need an new X-ray tent and dark-room tent, and will be glad if you can order them at once. Other things, of course, will be required, but I shall be able to deal better with our wants next week.

Many beds were broken, and many small comforts blown away and spoiled. It was really sad to see our beautiful comfortable camp, of which we are all so proud such a wreck.

Sister Maitland arrived yesterday. The syringes she brought with her were hailed with delight, as there was scarcely more than one whole syringe left in the place after the disaster.

We are all proud to say that we admitted five patients this morning—we were not *quite* ready for them but we managed, and tonight we are ready for twenty more, and are really a hospital again.

You will be pleased to know that the whole unit worked so admirably that it is hardly fair to specify names of those who excelled; but I, personally, feel deeply indebted to Miss Tubb, who fed the unit luxuriously; Miss Lindsay, who made lunches for the patients on their departures; Miss Greenlees, who was used everywhere; Sister Saunders, who, as always, is a tower of strength; and Miss Brown, who discovered and put out a threatened fire. The sisters worked hard for their patients' safety, and everybody did whatever offered and never a grumble was heard.

Since the collapse of the tents, the *bolnichars* have been beyond praise. It is they who have done all the erection of the wards and the mending of the torn tents. Nikola, the theatre *bolnichar*, saved practically everything in his theatre (which he loves as if it were his child), only a few glass dishes being broken, and then he mended the tent itself, and today, he proudly polished the drums to make it a theatre to rejoice our hearts.

In fact, I am proud of my unit, and think you will be the same.　(Sgd.)　　　　　　　　　　Mary de Garis.

Shortly after the date of this unit's removal upcountry in the wake of the Serbian Army, the following letter, which bears witness to its efficiency, was received from the Red Cross Commissioner in Salonika:

British Salonika Force, 3rd March 1919.

Dear Mrs. Hunter,—I am sure it will be of great interest to you to refer to the 3rd Supplement of the *London Gazette* of Tuesday, 21st January 1919 (published on Wednesday, 22nd January 1919), in which appears the dispatch of General Sir George F. Milne. K.C.B., D.S.O., the General Officer Commanding-in-Chief, British Salonika Force, dated General Headquarters. 1st December 1918.

In this dispatch the Commander-in-Chief reviews the operations of the British Army in Macedonia from the 1st October 1917 to the 1st December 1918, and in the course of his report he inserted the following paragraph, which I am sure will be very pleasing to your committee, namely:

I desire to take this opportunity of expressing my admiration of the work of the Scottish Women's Hospitals Organisations serving with the Serbian Army.

With kind regards, yours sincerely

　(Sgd.)　　　　　　　　　　H. Fitzpatrick.

Lieut.-Colonel. Commissioner

Mrs. James T. Hunter.

Chairman, Scottish Women's Hospitals for Foreign, Service, 2 St. Andrew Square, Edinburgh.

LETTER FROM A PATIENT AT OSTROVO

In my thirty-eight years of life I never had an opportunity to be in hospital and estimate the value of hospital service except now in Scottish Women's Hospital in Ostrovo. The work and the services and self-sacrifice of this patriotic and hospitable people we cannot sufficiently repay nor reward. The Director of the Hospital is Dr. de Garis, who is in charge of the whole hospital and its personnel. Miss Dr de Garis is a woman of medium build, physically well developed, energetical, and of serious look. Her every look, her every step, is of great importance and significance. You could see her every morning going over the hospital area and inspecting some swamps, which she formerly ordered to be levelled with earth.

A few minutes after, you see her in a hospital circle, and so on. until the visit of the patients commences. There is no nook in a hospital where she does not see it, or looks into, with the assistance of her true and worthy sisters, who with motherly care look for Serbian soldiers. After 8 o'clock commences the morning visit of patients. She steps into her ward, and with mild and courteous tone goes to every patient, and with smile on her face asks in Serbian, '*Kako vi? Boli glava, noga, ruka grudi,*' and as a rule always questions the patient what was he complaining of when he was first admitted to hospital.

Every patient answers promptly her questions just the way he feels, and she understands everything that soldiers tell her in Serbian. During the visit a sister is always present with her, in order that she may know by her prescription what medicine to give to the patient. The visit usually lasts till 12 o'clock. At 12 the bugler sounds for lunch, and Dr. de Garis, with her sisters, goes for lunch.

After lunch there should be rest for her, but, being brave among the braves, she avoids it, and with book on her table and knitting in her hands she reads her book and knits her socks. She does two works in one and the same time. If there is urgent case for an operation, which she always performs with skill, alertness, and success, she immediately leaves her book and drops her knitting, going quickly to the operating theatre. If new patient comes to the hospital, she never lets him wait five minutes unless she examines him. The sisters are detailed one in each ward on day duty, and one to four wards on night duty, with the addition of several orderlies.

In my ward was on day duty Sister ——. She rises at 6.30 in the morning. After her breakfast she goes immediately to pick flowers and wild roses. She comes afterwards to our ward with flowers in her hand, greeting us with good morning, and asking every patient how he slept, and patients promptly responding to her, 'Dobro, Sestra.'

Now begins her work. She opens the closet with medicines. and gives his own to every patient. Then she goes on with dressing of patients from the surgical operations, uttering and chatting with patients in Serbian, which she cannot yet distinctly pronounce. When she is about ready with her work it is 12 o'clock. In the interval the patients are always asking her for cigarettes, chocolate, and postcards. And you must believe that there is not a single patient that our good sister would not satisfy with whatever is possible.

For several days I was watching the sister, how she takes out of her ward one of our seriously ill patients supporting him under his left arm and giving him her umbrella to support himself with his right arm, walking with him in the shade that the great big trees in hospital area are giving us. Aware of how long this walk should last, she carries the pillow under her left arm, and only looks for suitable place and then puts her pillow on the ground, resting his head easily on the pillow. Then she sits to his left, asking him how does he feel. The same is with able Sister ——, for whom I have never enough praise.

She is giving so many sacrifices in ministering to our patients and otherwise that we must really admire her. I never expected to have such a treatment in Macedonia. Besides her nursing work she devotes most of her time to seriously ill cases, and finds for every one of them a word of spiritual comfort. This is what puts her in the rank of foremost nursing sisters. Having been in Serbia. Miss —— knows the Serbs and their thorny path through which they have gone, and that is why she can speak to Serbian patients heart to heart. It is impossible for me to write about all sisters, because I don't know their names in order to mention them all. But to be fair with them and not wanting to go into long discussions.

I must say for all we know, that they are worthy daughters of the great English race, conscious of their work and duty. They fully merit to be called sisters, and real sisters indeed, because our born sisters or mothers could not have so much patience and endurance to look over and minister to the Serbian soldier. All soldiers that were in this hospital for treatment, and with

299

whom I came in contact, and those that are here now, have only words of praise for the excellent treatment they have received at Scottish Women's Hospital.

I am convinced that these services rendered to our patients by lady doctors and sisters of the Scottish Women's Hospital shall remain deeply engraved into the hearts of mine and my war comrades as a remembrance and appreciation, which shall incite the later generations to reverence for what the Scottish Women have done for the Serbs, in the hour of their great need.

I will say once more, praise to the brave Scottish Women!

Sergt.-Maj. Milan Lubuvitch,
(300 2 Bat. Sect, post No. 36.)

"Praise to the brave Scottish Women!" But they do not want our praise. They have gained the love of Serbia, and as though the long years she remembers the sons who suffered and died for her in that last victorious struggle, she sees at their side the devoted, the tender-hearted, the brave the indomitable women that Britain had sent her.

And Ostrovo—can they ever forget Ostrovo? The scattered village, the lake with its circle of bare and rocky mountains, the camp in a fold of the hills, the trees round it, and the spring of fresh water beside it: the sad but absorbing work in operating-tent, the anxious watching in the wards, the ambulance cars ploughs their way through the sand or bumping and boiling the rocky tracks; the "hairpin bends" on the Drina, the flies at Skotchivar, the glare of the sun on the sand, the lashing rain, the delight in the cooled air, the boom of the guns, the sound of the fiddle brought from Salonika, the dance, the glorious camaraderie—there are women today in Australia and Britain who can never forget Ostrovo.

CHAPTER 3

The Transport Columns

From September 1916 to September 1918 the Serbian Army was waging war against the Bulgars in the Moglena Mountains. It is no country to fight in.

> Even with unlimited transport of all kinds, and men to get it up to the fighting line, it would be difficult to guarantee the armies against either scarcity of ammunition or food. And the Serbs had no such abundance. The way they have fought is magnificent—stupendous. But it has meant an untold amount of extra exposure and suffering. . . . What the Serbs have been through has to be told to be credited. All honour to a brave race.[1]

In transport of all kinds they were limited, but of motor ambulances they had none at all. The wounded were carried to the dressing-stations and hospitals and to the railway stations on their way to Salonika, in stretchers slung on either side of mules. The weary journey along the desperate mountain roads would often take hours. It is appalling to think what many a wounded man must have suffered on these journeys.

The Transport Column of the Scottish Women under Mrs. Harley was the only one working in these mountains for the Serbs. It arrived in Salonika shortly before Dr. Bennett's Unit in August 1916, and until the following January was encamped on the shores of Lake Ostrovo. In January 1917 Mrs. Harley resigned her post as Head of the Transport Column to do relief work in Monastir, and the column thereafter was attached to the Ostrovo Unit, under Miss Bedford. Miss Bedford tells the story of the year's work from September 1916 to August 1917.

---

1. *At the Serbian Front in Macedonia.*

During the past year the work of the M.T.Ambulance Section[2] has been as varied as it has been strenuous, and almost every sample of bad road has been experienced.

In their journeys for wounded, the ambulances have struggled and skidded on the steepest mountain gradients, and in the worst possible weather. The little vans (when plying for hospital provision) have laboured and stuck in unconquerable mud. There have been long, sad journeys to Salonika, bearing the remains of some dead hero to his last resting-place, and there has been happy ones, when sister, and orderlies going home on leave have been carried to their port of embarkation. And we find that with every journey, our respect for the 'Ford' has increased.

In September 1916 there were five ambulances, one lorry, and a touring-car attached to the hospital at Ostrovo. Although the actual distance covered and the number of patients carried, at the time, does not compare with the work of the Transport Column in the early months of the following year (after we moved forward), yet the roads were much more difficult, and the patients were nearly all desperately bad cases.

Our ambulances and those working under Mrs. Harley (which later did splendid work) ran over the same ground, bringing patients from dressing-stations, 14 or 15 kilometres up the mountains to our hospital and carrying convalescents to the various evacuating hospitals along the line of railway. In those days our beasts lay over quite recently fought over. Enormous shell-holes the way—piles of ammunition, used and unused, and many dead beasts. Amongst all the battle-leavings I know of no sadder sight than to meet the appeal in the eyes of a fallen horse in his last hours.

The comforts at these dressing-stations were not many, but the patients, when they arrived on mules from the front, either in pannier saddles or hammocks slung either side of the animal, were rested and fed: the straw upon which they were laid in the tents looked clean and their wounds were always carefully and skilfully dressed. The remarkable courage and chivalry of the Serbian soldier was often displayed on these ambulance journeys. He would endure pain and cold without a murmur,

---

2. Attached to the Ostrovo Unit. From Jan. 1917 moved with the unit that had been under Mrs. Harley.

and after a journey of intense torture, over broken and jolting ground, he would smilingly thank the chauffeur for her careful driving. Indeed, the Serbian soldier is a most lovable person, simple in character, is courageous in ruling his own spirit as he is in storming a mountain, full of faith, and with the heart of a child. The Hospital Sisters always said they were just like big children to nurse, and when the pain was at its worst their cry was invariably for their *micas* (mothers).

In those first days we had no facilities for mending the cars and no covering for them or for the 'spares,' which on arrival. I found in packing-case cupboard, standing in the open. After fruitless appeals for wood, in many directions, I finally thought of our commanding officer, a Serbian colonel with a reputation for organisation. His reply was characteristic. He sent an order for our lorry to be sent to his office next day, and in due time it returned with a generous supply of wood.

Then a tarpaulin was found, and a shelter was raised, raised, sufficient to cover three cars, with more cupboards her 'spares' and tools. Later we enlarged the structure and closed it in with walls of flattened petrol tins, and in the sun it shone like silver and was an object of much pride and of great comfort. The colonel's thoughtfulness a so provided us with a chauffeur and mechanic whom he secured from his brother (who was a general in Salonika), so that he might lend him to us.

Thus the nucleus of a garage was begun, and we were able to do our own small repairs. Here it will be fitting to render tribute to the unfailing help of the British Army Service Corps, several of whose camps were close, to our hospital. We have to thank them for keeping our cars on the roads in those first trying times, and also for much kindness then and since.

On Christmas Day the Serb chauffeurs and the hospital carpenter gave us a special *slava* or feast, for which they made elaborate preparations, where they displayed the truest hospitality. Having occasion to visit the garage before it was light. I found it illumined by an enormous fire at which a whole lamb was being roasted. Guyo was turning the spit and the other chauffeur was basting the carcase out of a petrol tin dish containing a strange fatty mixture.

They rose with the Serbian Christmas greeting 'The Christ is born.' They made me repeat the answer in Serbian, which means: 'I know that He is born"

When the roast was finished it was carried to their sleeping tent, and stood there to get cold At night it was cut up and served at a feast to which I and some of the chauffeurs were bidden. There was also a Christmas tree, upon which we were each represented by a carburettor. I was a sparking plug, and the carpenter was represented by a golden shaving hung on the topmost branch.

One dwells on the characteristics of these delightful people because one feels that they show what the Serbians are, and how entirely they deserve the help that we have given them, and surely they stand in need of it. They have fought bravely, times without number, against appalling odds, until those who are left are worn out, body and spirit. Kaimatchalan, where hundreds of their dead and their enemies' dead lie buried, is an everlasting monument to their bravery and their endurance. One of the few really decisive battles in the war's history, it was won under conditions impossible to describe. They have suffered the disseminating ravage of disease, and separation from their families, with no word of them for years (such are the Bulgars' cruel restrictions in Serbia). These sufferings truly have been forced upon them, but the spirit in which they have been endured is theirs, and theirs alone; this and their trust and dependence upon the British are an eloquent appeal to every one of us to stand by and protect them.

On 15th January 1917 the Transport Column under Mrs. Harley (as was mentioned before) was transferred to Dr. Bennett's Unit, and was attached to a dressing-station about 60 kilometres from the hospital where we had first worked. We found three fairly able-bodied ambulances, one totally out of action, two vans, and a kitchen car (also temporarily out of action and unsuited to the roads in that part of the country). The latter was subsequently converted into a van capable of carrying sitting cases, or material, and it proved most useful. One of the Ford vans we sent to Ostrovo. We had three more ambulances sent up from there, and as soon as possible put the disabled one on the roads, so that we had seven in all. The colonel also placed (for several months) four Serbian ambulances and their drivers directly under my control.

Then began a very busy time. The sick and wounded (they

were mostly sick) came down in large numbers from the front in carts and on mules They would often arrive covered with snow and soaked to the skin, and there were many cases of frostbite

Our (return) journey to the Evacuation Hospital near the line was about 34 kilometres, and sometimes the cars did four journeys in the day. There was never a day off, only half a day very occasionally. Rain and snow alternated, and the girls would come home with, icicles hanging to their eyes and all round their necks. Owing to a scarcity of paraffin and other causes there was no stove in the mess or sleeping tents, but they would cheerfully thaw themselves at the open trench fire in the camp kitchen, and after supper would fill their hot-water bottles and jump into bed, often with the snow drifting in under their tent flaps. Yet I never once heard them grumble. They were ready for the roads every morning soon after dawn, and the more driving they had the better pleased they were.

The task of making a garage more portable than the 'silver palace' we had left behind at the hospital then began, and the hunt for wood had to be resumed. The trees for many miles round our camp had been cut down by the troops, and it was with great difficulty that even firewood could be found. However, at that time I had to visit Salonika on one of the periodical hunts for 'motor spares,'[3] and I happened to mention the needed wood in the presence of a naval officer, who had once spent a few days with Mrs. Harley, and who knew the work of the Transport Column. He immediately spoke to his captain, with wonderful results.

The model erection which for a time graced our camp we owed to the kindness of this officer, but, alas! it was scarcely finished when our marching orders came, and the column was moved, with the dressing-station, across the river, and there, profiting by our recent experience, we raised a still better and yet more portable shelter for our cars. We were then in the proud position of being able to lend some of our precious wood to finish the hospital kitchen and to make a locked store, as well as ward screens, and even shafts for the Serbian horse-carts (which were often in the wars), to say nothing of seats for the mess tent.

3. Miss Bedford was known from one end of Serbia to the other as "Miss Spare parts," due to her search for motor accessories!

About this time our work slackened. We were given a long, tedious run of 60 kilometres (return journey) over a road so rough that our mortality for 'springs' increased by leaps and bounds, and springs in those days were unprocurable. But necessity knows no law. The ambulances had to be kept on the roads, and it meant journeys of 300 kilometres to Salonika, and then unending difficulties. But we felt we must uphold the garage tradition. No order for carrying wounded could ever be refused. I am glad to say that it never was, except on one occasion, when the weather rendered the roads impassable.

Just before we left this camp there were several hostile air raids, and bombs were dropped unpleasantly close to the hospital. The cars were always sent out to search for casualties, which, alas! we always found and were able to render timely aid.

In April we had a move to a far less picturesque site in a barren, sandy valley entirely shut in by hills. It was intolerably hot, and as the place had been an old horse camp the flies were unendurable. Rations were sometimes difficult to get, and the bread was often mouldy. Our ambulance, now numbering fourteen, had a good stand and the workshop and store were conveniently placed, and our facilities and arrangements for repairing the cars were much improved.

But for many months our eyes had been set on the hills from whence the wounded came; however, the military authorities did not consider the roads fit for ambulances, especially as the cases were then mostly light and could travel without discomfort by cart. Early in May we were ordered to run up to a dressing-station about eight kilometres from us, which had moved forward, and to which patients from three different sections of the front were received. It was, however, not considered worthwhile to move our camp for so short a distance, especially as when the loads were finished we should be running right on to the next ambulance at the very summit.

On 15th June we covered the whole distance for the first time. It would be difficult indeed to give a true idea of the beauty and interest of this journey. The road zigzags up the sides of the mountain a distance of about eighteen kilometres. From each 'hairpin bend' a different view of the country is obtained. At one point peak after peak, in bold, irregular outline, rises against a brilliant blue sky, and then as we turn, we find that we are facing deep dark gorges which seem to drop straight from the road we are on, almost out of sight. Then another turn brings us to more gentle slopes covered with undergrowth, until we reach the dressing-station (on the sides of a steep, pine-sheltered summit from which we now are to carry the patients).

In July the welcome orders came that we might move up the Transport Section to this fascinating spot.[4] The *Médecin-Chef* chose with me a site for our camp, and he did everything he possibly could to make us comfortable. The kitchen and mess room rose like magic in a single day, the work of his Serbian *bolnichars*, who were discharged soldiers. The kitchen, with its French fires, its primitive stone oven, its roof of pine branches, and its pretty cook (one of our Ostrovo orderlies), made a delightful picture.

Next to it was a small store built of pine logs, with a roof of branches covered with the same, which made it both cool and rainproof and the bower which served as a mess-room was made entirely of pine saplings and foliage closely interlaced, with the front fairly open and commanding a magnificent view towards Monastir. The only drawback to our new site was the distance from the garage, which made the supervision of the work somewhat difficult. But the Serbian mechanic is a conscientious worker, and I could always feel that he was to be trusted.

If the winter does not temporarily drive the column back to more sheltered quarters, the prospects of moving still farther forward are excellent, as the road to the dressing-station, about four kilometres nearer the firing-line, is rapidly being improved, and if this point is reached, the usefulness of the Transport Column will be much increased.

YELLAK, AUGUST 1917.

From August 1917 to September 1918, at which latter date the Serbian advance began, the column was stationed at Yellak high up in the mountains, on a spur of Kaimatchalan, where the Serbs built wooden huts for the whole party. Their work during this year was incessant. The cars were off the roads only two days throughout the winter. The nature of the roads was such that it is hard indeed to understand how the girl chauffeurs dared to take their cars over them—

---

4. Yellak.

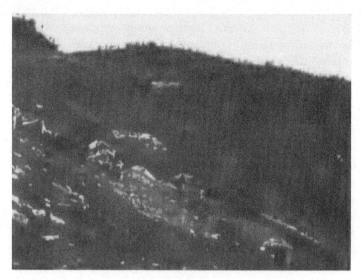

YELLAK

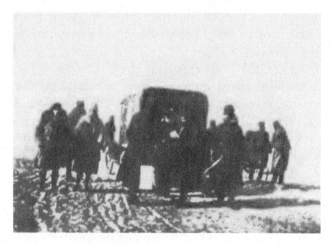

STARTING ON A COLD MORNING

narrow, steep paths, with deep precipices on the one hand and high cliffs on the other. Many women would find it in their hearts to envy the members of the Transport Column this year spent at Yellak, 5000 feet high

The huts were clustered together on the hillside, far from any other community, amidst wild and fascinating scenery. The work which occupied the girls daily called continuously for a display of high virtues, courage, endurance, and extreme gentleness. They lived physically and morally in a keen, bracing atmosphere. We read one of the diaries of the sorrow with which they moved on in September 1918 from their home on the mountain-side, though they were overjoyed to be accompanying the Serbs in their advance into their own country. Writing of the women of the Transport Column in Russia attached to the London Units, Dr. Inglis says:

> Their nerve never failed them, they never lost their courage, and they never forgot to be gentle.

The same is true of the members of this Transport Column in Macedonia.

During the year at Yellak the Scottish Women in their ambulances "scoured the country for wounded," and became well known along the mountain tracks, with their "hairpin bends." Stationed at each of these bends were old Serbian soldiers—*chichas* (uncles), as they were called—to control the traffic of the motors and ambulances nearing the corners. At first the *chichas* used green boughs, which were waved furiously in the air to warn the traffic. The boughs not proving very efficient, whistles were substituted, but with little improvement. The whistles of the exited old men were heard continuously along the mountain sides and lost all value to the approaching drivers. Boards painted red on one side and white on the other were ultimately chosen.

The *chichas* were devoted to the Scottish Women. One day, during the period the column was stationed at Yellak, one of the S.W.H. ambulances was stopped, when going up a steep path by the warning from the red board at the "hairpin bend." Behind the ambulance was a convoy of M.T. wagons toiling up the steep road, and this of course had also to halt. The old *chicha* vanished from his post for a moment behind a boulder, then appeared again with an old bully-beef tin, in which was arranged a bunch of wild flowers. This with great delight he presented to "the Goddess in the Car." It is not difficult to imagine the feelings of the M.T. men, who had had to pull up for this act of devotion, and would now have to spend several minutes restarting their wagons on this steep bend. However, it is good to hear the Tommies took it as a great joke, cheered the old *chicha*, helped to restart the S.W.H. ambulance, and then worked at their own.

The advance of the Serbian Army, beginning in the middle of September 1918 and culminating in their entry into Belgrade on 1st November, is one of the marvellous stories of the war. The quotations which follow from Miss Corbett's diary give us a vivid impression of the part which the Scottish Women took in this wonderful advance, and Miss Dillon, Head of the Transport since Miss Bedford had returned to Australia, takes up the story where Miss Corbett stops, and carries us right into Belgrade.

Nish, 22nd October 1918.

Dear Miss Ferguson,—We have had a most eventful month, and I cannot give you a better idea of it than by sending you extracts from Miss Corbett's diary, which she has kindly made for me.

On the whole, we have had a most successful trek. We have had to leave 2 cars on the way, and now have 14 out of our original 16, but the Serbs only have 5 out of 12, and the French 6 out of 20. The nearest M.T. Coy. is nearly a couple of hundred kilometres behind us.

We have had a great reception in all the towns, as the soldiers have told the women of 'their sisters,' and they hang wreaths ever the cars and give us fruit and flowers.

The health of the unit has been excellent up to here (Nish), but now four people have influenza, which is rampant in the country. We are stopping here for a little, and I hope that it will give them time to recover.

(Sgn.) Kathleen Dillon.

Yellak, Sunday, 15th September 1918.—It was indeed the offensive yesterday, and all the guns must haw been going after all. Colonel Petrovitch (Medical Chief of our Army) came over from H.Q. this morning to tell us that Sokal and Dobrapolje had both fallen at seven o'clock, and we heard afterwards that we've taken 1000 prisoners and a great many guns. Wonderful news, indeed, for now that first and worst mountain barrier has fallen so quickly, it means that a big advance is certain. The

Serbs have waited so long, just on three years of exile now—three years in many cases without so much as a postcard from home, and a Serb loves his home almost better than a Frenchman does.

It's rather pathetic the way they have idealised their country: there, there are perfect roads, we are assured, as we bump along over these, and large gardens bright with flowers even under the snow and magnificent houses, and no mountains at all! And we, who remember 'real Serbia.' rather wonder It they'll have a horrid disillusionment, or be perfectly content when they get back to their smiling and delightful but certainly roadless, land. Anyhow, they're very radiant today; as I went down the road this morning an old fellow coming up on an ammunition cart leant over the edge till I thought he'd fall out, shouting, '*Sestra, Sestra! Sma dobra, Sestra!*' (Sister, it is well); and there was a ring in his voice that brought a lump to one's throat.

Tuesday, 17th September.—Good news again today. The Second Army took Koziak last night, the last of the enemy's defences really this side of Prilep and the Babuna, and our army has advanced 10 kilometres in some places. The Serbs have taken 4000 prisoners altogether (they were coming down to H.Q. to be counted all day) and 51 guns, and if only this perfect weather holds there's no saying where we may get to!

All went down to Danube II 6.15 this morning. They'd 120 wounded in, but M. G—— sent down a dozen of his Fiat ambulances that take eight men each, and M. W—— a lot of Fords, and they cleared them out, so only three of our cars had to go back there after lunch, and a couple to Drina III. Drina II. to which we've been attached for over a year now, moved this morning early, to away beyond Milutina Kosa, where there are no roads at all, and we're left rather stranded, as they cherished and fed us, and brought us wood and water. They've left us a couple of men though, so we shall manage all right.

Wednesday, 18th September.—Packed till 10 a.m. in expectation of a move, when I started for Drina III—got back at 2.15 and lunched hastily, then down to Danube II, getting home after seven—too late and dark to do anything more in the way of preparations.

Friday, 20th September.—Tremendous uprooting all day: one

gets so firmly anchored in a year; and one can carry so awfully little in a Ford on these roads. We're to take a haversack each, and bed.; and bedding tomorrow, as well as part of our stores and part of the garage stuff and the tents. Sister and Kent the cook are being left behind for a day or two with one of the garage men, and are to get our kit-bags and things sent on in M. G——'s big cars, which will no doubt always be taking patients back from whichever dressing-station we run to.

Saturday, 21st September (Nobody knows where)—Off at last on the longed-for move forward, and it's really very sad, when the moment comes, to say goodbye to our log huts and well-known mountainous land.

Sunday, 22nd September (Miletznitza).—Did one run back to Danube I (some of them did two), but must of the wounded were light cases and sent away in carts or on their own feet. Got orders at midday to come on here, so came, arriving about four o'clock—15 kilos farther forward. This is a desperate army to keep up with! We've no news at all, but they must be advancing at a pretty brisk pace. We've installed ourselves in very clean Bulgar huts, and found three large vats of Bulgar petrol, but goodness knows when we'll see the rest of our unit or possessions again.

Wednesday, 25th September (Belavoda).—M'Caw went back from here this morning to try and collect our various possessions, which have got badly scattered between this and Yellak, nobody having foreseen a trek of this rapidity.

Up at five and helped to carry the dressing-station, so didn't get in here till midday. It's about 25 kilos (the same as yesterday's run) by the road, but not nearly as much on the map—zigzag up one side of the mountain and zigzag down the other. We'd been promised good roads after Dunje, but I suppose it depends on what you call 'after.' This one's very steep and very deep sand in several places, where sticking is quite inevitable; but there's plenty of traffic on the road, so one just waits till a sufficient crowd collects to shove one. At the dressing-station found forty Italian and Roumanian prisoners left behind here sick, in a wretched shed, and in a bad state of starvation and rags, so our nine cars took twenty-seven of them back to Dunje.

Thursday, 26th September (Prilep).—The Serbs are on the point of taking Veles, 60 kilos beyond Prilep, and surely this is being one of the epic advances of history? In our cars we can't keep up with the army, which is marching and fighting at the same time!

We've emerged from our five days struggle in the wilderness, breathless but triumphant. I'm very glad we had that 'trek,' though it's a comfort to see main roads and civilisation again. If the weather had broken up there in the hills and turned the sand to mud we'd never have got either back or forward again.

Friday, 27th September (Babuna)—No patients ready till midday, so worked on the cars. Then did two journeys to Prilep, 15 kilos away; trundled a borrowed back axle back for '19' and set our after the others about 6.30, up over the Babuna—and down and down and down—hairpin bend after hairpin bend, a perfect nightmare of them, till at last I came on the column (11 p.m.) drawn up by the roadside, asleep either in their cars or in their beds in the ditch—the dressing-station slumbering around them. All the grass and scrub ahead of us seemed to be on fire, roaring and leaping tongues of flame everywhere— wonderful sight!

Saturday, 28th September (Veles).—On, very early this morning, to the village that had been indicated to us; had just pitched our tents—and were very pleased with ourselves—beside trees and a stream when a man came along with orders that we were to move right on here—a tremendous trek for the dressing-station after its hard work, fully 40 kilos, the men and most of the officers on foot, and all the staff on mule-back. Worrall went straight back to Prilep with three wounded who turned up from somewhere, and I took three sick that we found in an ox-cart back to Igvor. It's one of the loveliest towns I've ever seen; white houses with brown-tiled roofs climbing irregularly up the banks of the broad and placid Vardar River, thickly embowered in its trees, and with the usual graceful minarets springing up lightly here and there.

We've camped on a somewhat squalid spot, just above the big barracks that the Germans have been using as a hospital, a perfect building for it, with big rooms, light and airy; but the dressing-stations have so little equipment that they can't do much till they get some of the hospitals up. The enemy only cleared out the night before last, so the station buildings are burning still, but the town seems all right. We hit off the main line north from Salonika here for the first time, and once they get the trains working on it again everything will be much easier.

Sunday, 29th September (Veles).—Took two Bulgars and a Frenchman back to Prilep, 60 kilometres and a six hours' journey, for though the road is broad and level till you come to the Babuna, it's horribly bumpy still. The poor Bulgars screamed the whole way, and I'd to stop several times to try and arrange their wounded legs better, but there's very little one can do; a bumpy road is bound to hurt fiendishly, however slowly one goes. They've still only a very messy dressing-station squatted in a corner of the barracks at Prilep, so the patients have another long day's journey on to Banitza in M. G——'s cars.

Monday, 30th September.—A beautiful day again, to our great relief, and the river, with the trees beyond it and the hills behind, looked very lovely in the rain-washed air. It is pleasant, too, not to be breathing dust for an hour or two. Most of us cleaned our cylinder heads. Three of the cars were ordered off at an hour's notice to take a doctor and three orderlies to Koumanovo away beyond Skoplje, 100 kilometres off at least. There were no orders for the rest of us till 9 o dock tonight when two of us were sent off with an imbecile guide to look for some slightly wounded somewhere in this tortuous town. Heaven knows where we drove, but when it came to a sort of narrow gutter up a precipitous cliff between two blank walls, a place it would take a clever mule to negotiate, we struck and came home. They can be fetched far more suitably by hand tomorrow.

They say Bulgaria has surrendered unconditionally, and that terms are being arranged in Paris. Of course Germany and Austria remain, but it spells triumph for the Serbs at last. Everybody's crowding into the town tonight, and at every turn you're greeted exultantly and your hand wrung by the chancest acquaintance. It is very glorious for them. They've had an awfully strenuous time, of course, and not much to eat, but they aren't feeling it yet. I said to one of the hospital orderlies yesterday that he must have had very hard work. 'There is much to do,' he said; 'but work is not hard when one is going home!' And that is the feeling everywhere.

Tuesday, 1st October (Skoplje).—Off at 8.30 this morning by a disappointing road, hilly at first but afterwards broad and level, along the fertile Vardar valley, and maddeningly bumpy; it was a case of low speed nearly all the way, into holes and over bumps. There were several bridges destroyed, one big one still burning merrily, but by sending a much-amused Macedonian to walk backwards and forwards through the water at several points we found a quite passable ford.

The inhabitants have come out tonight in quite sufficient quantities to relieve our minds, and the electric street lamps installed by the Germans are twinkling cheerfully. It's a queer sort of town, this ancient capital of Serbia, with two rows of big gaunt houses along by the river, which is spanned by handsome bridges. one rather mean cobbled street of shops, and the old part huddled up behind, with only a few minarets to relieve the squalor of its blank walls. Turkish customs do not make for cheerful streets, as the gardens are all carefully screened and almost no windows face the outer world.

Wednesday 2nd October (Koumanovo).—Went up to the citadel with Miss Dillon this morning to ask about the road, and were told by high authorities that we might start whenever we liked, but the cavalry were starting at 12, so perhaps we'd like to go with them. We searched wildly for petrol, and at last found a small keg of benzol at the station. I'm beginning to hate the sight of kegs of benzol, it makes cranking the cars *such* a business; but its better than not running at all. and we've lived on loot ever since we left Yellak, having outstripped all the other cars and official supplies.

At midday the cavalry, mounted on sturdy little horses, started with their band playing but in full battle array of shrapnel helmets and arms. We set out cheerfully after them, and soon overtook them, then got in here just behind the scouts, the rest of the regiment coming along soon afterwards, a very pretty sight, played through the town by their band on white horses, pacing five abreast. H.Q. arrived tonight, I believe, and we saw three Bulgar officers with an armed retinue riding in for a *pourparler.* They really do seem to have capitulated on the whole, but there are little parties of them still scrapping.

This is a dear little town on a stream, with poplar trees and minarets, and open booths and Turkish inhabitants, but there seemed no clean houses in it so we've pitched the tents in the open again, and 'the open' is all rather bare and burnt up.

Saturday, 5th October (Koumanovo).—Off at 7 a.m. and home 9.30 p.m.—driving steadily the whole time, and accomplished 120 miles. What a country! Coll. Petrovitch told us to send three cars to look for patients in a couple of villages where he believed there were dressing-stations, and to find out which side of Vranja the enemy is, with a view to moving there to-morrow! We drew the first village blank, but a little farther on found some wounded Austrians sheltering in the abandoned lorry; they'd been there for three days without food, they said, and looked pretty miserable. Ellis took them back, and Miss Dillon and I went on.

I picked up a very ill Serb on the road, and we also gave lifts to several ambulance people plodding frontwards. It was a beastly day, a bitter wind in the morning and heavy rain from 11 o'clock on. The road is awfully bumpy, straight and flat, but innocent of metal as far as we probed it through the mud, and full of holes. Blocked, too, today with every sort of traffic: dozens of big guns, some cavalry, a whole infantry division, three dressing-stations on the move, and strings and strings of pack ponies, army carts, native carts—but we'd the honour of being the only motors fools enough to try it! There are at least a dozen bridges broken; one big one necessitates fording a river just deep enough for the cars, and the little ones also present a pleasant variety of obstacles, with the one unchanging feature of MUD.

We had to be shoved a lot, often empty, and it's going to be quite impossible tomorrow with loaded cars, I fear. We were lured on and on with rumoured dressing-stations just ahead, until we finally got to Vranja itself, which the enemy evacuated last night. The Bulgars have really capitulated now, but the Austrians and a couple of German regiments are still scrapping a bit as they retire.

Vranja is the first town we've been allowed to call 'real Serbia,' and the people came rushing out joyfully to greet us, with wreaths of flowers, marigolds and love-lies-bleeding, to hang on the radiator caps. All the cavalry horses were wearing wreaths too. and flags out everywhere, and this wretched weather spoiling it all! We found Danube II just arriving at the big Barracks Hospital,[1] so I deposited my sick man there. There were some Serbian sisters, kindly looking women, and a certain amount of equipment left by the Bulgars, and not too many patients, so we didn't suggest bringing any back here, the odds seeming about even on our getting back over the river after this rain. As a matter of fact it wasn't as bad as we'd expected, and seemed not to have risen at all, but some of the other mud-holes were pretty hopeless.

Monday, 7th October (Vranja).—We've got the empty top storey of such an attractive house, with a vine wandering out on a quaint wooden erection ever so far in front of its door, and a delightful well with a roof over it and a big wheel, and our welcome was even more floral and effusive today, but, alas! it still rains and ruins everything.

Tuesday, 8th October (Vranja).—We passed Vranski Banja, where the Ostrovo S.W.H. is supposed to be going, so turned aside to see that fashionable health resort with its hot springs smelling strongly of sulphur; but there's nothing fashionable today about the pretty little wooded valley with its couple of big boarding-houses empty and deserted.

The river was full of peasant women washing clothes in the hot water—such pretty, graceful creatures. Their clothes are beautiful too, coloured kerchiefs on their heads and a little rough brown *coatee* over the long very full striped petticoat that swings like a kilt when they walk; and the stripes are such glorious colours, vermilion and orange and black, as a rule, but there are blues and greens and purples too.

This is really the beginning of the home-coming, and we gave lifts to a group of very radiant men this morning, going back to their '*Komandos*' after finding the families they'd had no news of for three years alive and well.

Friday, 11th October (Leskovatz).—Got in here at lunch-time, after 25 kilos of very bad roads, and our welcome was certainly amazing. We were literally fallen upon by the entire population,

---

1. Afterwards taken over by the Scottish Women's Hospital from Ostrovo.

had wreaths hung round our own necks as well as our cars, and an embracing crowd of women and girls surged up and down the town after us, imploring us to go and stay with them, to lunch with them then—at least to come home with them for just five minutes, that their aged mothers might see us. I heard an agonised voice from the midst of the crowd: 'Isn't it terrible to be Scotch just now? You do feel so embarrassed with a whole string of them hanging round your neck,' and I could but agree sadly.

They must have been awfully disappointed at even our best efforts at responsiveness. We had coffee in a small shop, breathed and leant heavily upon by several hundred excited spectators, the back rows mounted on tables and chairs, and finally sought refuge in the first empty house that presented itself—a dirty and dilapidated structure that harrowed our admirers terribly; but a boy with a bayonet guarded the entrance against most of them, and we got some prisoners to clean it up a bit. The soldiers seem to have let themselves go, about us, to some effect. I heard a most spirited description of us under shell fire being delivered in a shop the other day; the Charge of the Light Brigade simply wasn't in it!

We're almost the first cars in, as a matter of fact. We passed half a dozen broken down on the way, and another half-dozen have won through with H.Q. people, and so on, but we're the first unit, and congratulating ourselves heartily on getting all the cars along.

Met the *commissaire* of Danube II in the town, who said they'd a lot of wounded 13 kilometres away; so, having found a small quantity of benzol, we all went out and brought some of them in, but most came in ox-carts or walked.

Saturday, 12th October (Leskovatz)—Did one run to Danube II this morning, and found the school building here, where Morava II is established, quite full, so had to take my patients to another big building near. I went in with my stretchers to see how things were, and found the place simply awful; absolutely empty, not a bed, not a stretcher, not a cup of water—only a very little straw spread round the sides of the rooms, and the sick and wounded lying on it all mixed up together. Two wounded women in one crowded 'ward,' one with a fractured femur and one with a newborn baby that she didn't know in the least what to do with. No doctor, and no real orderlies, only a few flustered people from the town.

As very few cars could go this afternoon (petrol all finished), half a dozen of us went over to see what we could do—and found it precious little. We got the sick all upstairs, and the wounded all downstairs, and the women into a separate room; and we got more straw, and Miss Dillon got some Austrian prisoners; and the ladies from the town began to surge in. They brought cups and water-jugs, and plates and food, and a few beds, on to which we got the worst cases, with straw wrapped up in our mosquito nets as mattresses; but there are no blankets, and very few pillows, and it is terrible how little one can do with only one's hands and no appliances at all. The first time I went into one of the rooms a man greeted me eagerly with, 'An English Sister. Has the hospital come from Ostrovo, then?' And how heartily I wished it had.

We captured sister and Miss Munn for our annexe today, and they've done wonders there. We've got a lot more beds and mattresses, too, but of course until we get blankets the men can't be got out of their torn and bloody uniforms, and only half a dozen of them have been dressed today. Several legs and hands are looking pretty nasty tonight, and several temps, are alarmingly high, and of course they're nearly all in a good deal of pain and discomfort. Thank Heaven Drina III has arrived with two excellent surgeons and a lot of material.

It's awful how little one can do with no doctor to order treatments, nor appliances to carry them out. The ladies of the town are in too, it being Sunday. They've supplied the beds and the mugs, and as the patients are their own men, whom they haven't seen for three years, one can't interfere much; but it is distressing to see a 'head' with a high temp, lapping up *nakia* (potent plum brandy), or a 'chest,' whose life hangs by a thread, dragged out of his bed and his proper position to have his mattress exchanged for a better one.

They're nearly all doing extraordinarily well, though, and a Serb certainly has amazing recuperative powers. Two men died—a gangrenous leg that should have been amputated, and a sick man from upstairs; and some of the worst cases have rather gone to bits tonight, leaning very dolefully one against another, and wanting small attentions continuously—but the pluck of most of 'em's wonderful.

Wednesday, 16th October (Leskovatz).—Wire last night that that petrol had been sent off, and we were all to go to Nish, so we've danced on the doorstep all day, packed and ready to start, and now comes a circumstantial rumour that the petrol's coming by ox-cart and can't be here till tomorrow night.

Thursday, 17th October (Nish).[2]—Petrol arrived in ox-carts early this morning, so the rest of us came on here, 45 kilometres of bumpy road, but dry again now after several summer days, and even the river gave almost no trouble. They say it's never been so low at this season before.

Found ourselves established in excellent quarters here, an ex-German club, empty but clean and airy. The others went off to Prohuplje directly after lunch for patients, and I did five 8-kilometre journeys round about the town, emptying one local hospital into another. Nish's a much more magnificent city than our memory had painted it. Three years ago, arriving without pause from London, and finding ourselves knee-deep in mud, it struck us as more like a south of Ireland village than anything else; whereas now, after a lengthy sojourn in Macedonia, it really seems a very fine modern town set in the midst of a wide plain.

Friday, 18th October (Nish).—Fetched patients from Prohuplje this morning. 60 kilometres there and back of rather nice rolling open country, with very pretty villages here and there, and sharp blur hills a long way off.

Saturday, 19th October (Nish).—To Prohuplje this morning, but found on arrival that I'd a ball race badly gone, so had to come home on Mac's bus, and send Voyoslav out to mine. Breakages are serious matters nowadays, but we've really had wonderful luck so far, considering the roads. We've got fourteen of our original sixteen here safely, and M. W——'s only got SIX out of his twenty—and there's no M.T. Company within 100 miles of us now.

Miss Dillon takes us into Belgrade:

---

2. See letter from Miss Dillon, at the start of these diary extracts, written from Nish.

We worked at Nish for ten days, and then went on to Krushevatz. Fighting was really over, though Krushevatz had gas shells dropped in it, and there were deaths from the results while we were there. The people had had to live in their cellars for some days. We got into Belgrade on 11th November, the army having reached it on the 1st, fourteen out of our original sixteen cars completing the journey.

And so we finished our trek of 740 kilometres, from one end of Serbia to the other. Our army gave us a very flattering mention in dispatches; the Prince Regent reviewed us and presented medals; and now we are waiting in a little town in Hungary till the right time comes to be demobilised.

7 St. Leonard s Terrace, Chelsea,
11th June 1919.

Extract From a Letter to the Committee.—

On my arrival in Belgrade last December, it was most gratifying to hear the universal praises of our hospitals, and especially of Miss Dillon's Transport. They earned undying fame for their splendid work in the final offensive.—Believe me, yours always gratefully,

E. Haverfield.

Ordre

Iière Armée
Etat Major.
Adj. No. 41163.

General Headquarters, Novi Sud.
19th January 1919.

From the Commander-in-Chief of the Serbian Army

Miss Kathleen Dillon, Commandant of the Scottish Women's Transport Column, who has undeniably earned the crown of success for the very heavy work of her column, and by showing under all circumstances a splendid example.

For these services and her fine actions I cite Miss Dillon at the Order of the Army.

The Voivode Commanding the 1st Serbian Army.

(Sgd.)   Boiovitch.

Ordre

Iière Armée Serbe
Etat Major.
Adj. No. 41163.

General Headquarters, Novi Sud.

19th January 1919.

From the Commander-in-Chief of the Serbian Army

The Motor Transport Column of the Scottish Women attached to the 1st Serbian Army under the command of Miss Kathleen Dillon, which before the beginning of the offensive was encamped near Yellak, helped with the evacuation of the wounded and sick from the farthest advanced dressing-stations up to Skotchivar and Banitza by a road frequently exposed to the enemy's fire, which was also very difficult, steep, and mountainous.

The strenuous task of this column having redoubled at the commencement of operations, the evacuation of the wounded at Kust, Rachin Potok, and Poltchichte, in spite of constant obstructions on the road, was effected as usual and without interruption. At the time of a great and stupendous need the column went up to Poltchichte, passing through Gradeshnitza and afterwards on to Melnitza. As soon as the enemy had been driven over the Czerna, the first ambulance to ford this latter was one belonging to this column. The column afterwards passed on to Dunje, Bela Vodista Troiatsi, and arrived at Veles, where it accompanied the advance guard of the French cavalry, entering Koumanovo with that. Further, in spite of bad weather, which impeded the work, the members of the column surmounted all difficulties with right goodwill and cheerfulness. This splendid example of endurance, devotion, and goodwill has produced an excellent influence on our soldiers who were fortunate enough to witness it.

The journeys from Koumanovo to Vranja, Leskovatz, and Nish were very difficult: difficulties which had to be conquered by goodwill, energy, and courage. The column was never late.

For these splendid feats I cite the column at the Order of the Army.

The Voivode Commanding the 1st Serbian Army,

(Sgd.) Boiovitch.

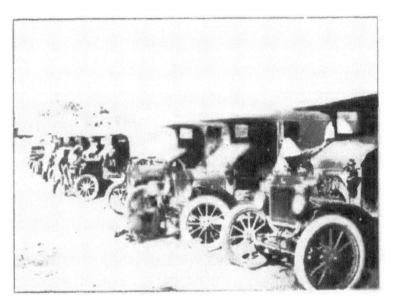

The Transport Column
"The column that was never late"

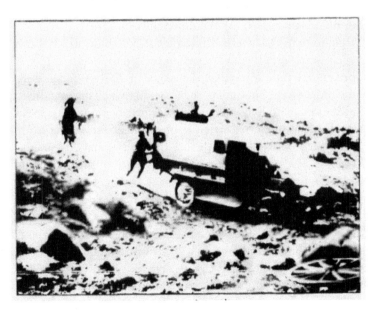

On the road to Dunje

THE STORY OF THE TRANSPORT COLUMN ATTACHED TO THE "ELSIE INGLIS" UNIT

The part played by this transport from the time it arrived at the camp until it rejoined the hospital at Sarajevo is given as follows by Miss Robinson, who succeeded Miss Geraldine Hedges as Chief Transport Officer when the latter was obliged to return home owing to severe and repeated attacks of malaria:

> Our official title was Motor Ambulance Section No. 8. and the section should have consisted of 8 ambulances, 1 Ford van, 3 touring-cars, and 11 Burford lorries. It was a great blow to us when the ship containing the 10 lorries and touring-car was torpedoed. The lorries and car were replaced, but arrived too late to be of any service.
>
> We settled into our camp near Dragomantsi on 1st April and soon got into full work. The primary purpose of the cars was, of course, to serve our own hospital, but in addition the ambulances went out every day and worked for all the dressing-stations of the three divisions of the 2nd Serbian Army—the Timok, Choumadia, and Jugo-Slav Divisions. These stations were scattered about all over the Mogleintsa valley and some of the roads—marked in red on our maps—were under fire from the Bulgarian batteries in the mountains.
>
> In the hot weather we had breakfast at 5.30 a.m. and the cars which were on duty kit at 6. and proceeded to the dressing-stations, where they worked all the morning. The wounded were brought down the mountains by mules, either to the first dressing-station or to a point where the road became practicable for a car. and our cars carried them to other dressing-stations, to our own Hospital, or to the big British General Hospitals at Vertekop. The drivers then had lunch with the Serbian Hospital Staff—it was particularly pleasant at Tressina and Kapiniani, where the tables were laid under shady trees and there always seemed to be a pleasant breeze.
>
> In the afternoon every one slept and work was resumed about 3 o'clock. The driving at night was rather difficult; it was, of course, forbidden to carry lights, and the narrow roads were blocked by endless processions of hay or provision carts and the long convoys of A.S.C. Ford vans carrying munitions to the foot of the mountains, whence they were carried to the

trenches by mules. It was interesting work, the men were pathetically grateful (gratitude seems to be a Serbian characteristic), and the sitting case on the front seat with the driver would begin eagerly to tell her about his family, and on the slightest provocation would produce the photographs of all his relatives and insist on her looking at them.

Later on, to prevent the daily waste of time and petrol in getting to the distant dressing-stations, a small advanced camp was formed at Kosturian; two or three charming mud huts were put up for us by the Serbs, and we pitched our tents in a mulberry grove. Though very hot and dusty, this was a very pleasant camp, and those of us who were not on duty were kept busy entertaining the visitors. They also took us to one or two of the performances at the regimental field theatres, and one was driven to the conclusion that every Serb is an actor by instinct.

During the influenza epidemic the ambulances were very busy: on one occasion four cars were on duty continuously from 7 a.m. on one day to 7 a.m. the next. The drivers came in full of energy, and were bitterly disappointed at being ordered to bed.

All through the summer, preparations were being pushed forward for the autumn offensive, and there were fresh rumours every day as to when it would begin. The Serbs were full of hope and enthusiasm, but later on there was some apprehension lest something should go wrong at the eleventh hour, and a comparatively small, though important advance was all that most people dared hope for. It meant so much to them, and their enthusiasm and excitement when they succeeded beyond their wildest dreams is indescribable. The officers said that it would have been quite impossible to stop the men if they had tried: the one cry was, 'Send us munitions—never mind the food, bring shells;' and the British A.S.C. men and the French lorry drivers toiled indefatigably day and night to keep them supplied.

When the offensive began, seven ambulances went over Kaziak with the Second Army and accompanied them (over roads which could only be regarded as a bad practical joke) through Kavadar, Negotin, and Slitip to Veles, where they met the hospital and the rest of the Transport. The S.W.H. suffered a good deal from lack of warm clothes and of food, in spite of the chivalrous efforts of some of the Serbian officers—notably Colonel (afterwards General) Zhievanovitch. Two drivers were also sent back seriously ill to Salonika.

In the meantime the rest of us broke up the camp at Vibliani, and after a short and useful though uncomfortable pause at Donii Pojar (there were millions of flies and five dead horses or mules within smelling distance!) proceeded to Monastir by road. At this point the weather broke and we camped at Vertekop for a few days in seas of mud. Then began the unforgettable journey through Serbia. We passed over the famous Babuna Pass, where St. Sava appeared to lead the Serbian troops to victory, and all the way in both directions there were endless streams of French lorries, Serbian carts. A.S.C. Ford vans, Serbian and French infantry, and Bulgarian prisoners finding their own way to the rear.

At Skoplje we all met again, but after a few days, leaving the hospital and a few cars behind, the ambulance section went forward with the headquarters of the Second Army. We went through Serbia to Uzice on the Bosnian frontier, seeing the most indescribably beautiful scenery and the most heartrending scenes of human misery. The mountains were clothed in all the glory of their autumn colours, the sun shone on the snow-sprinkled peaks and the rivers dashing below, and along the muddy roads trudged weary old-young men, who, their constitutions undermined by malaria, were now collapsing under the strain of the campaign or falling hopeless victims to the influenza epidemic.

At Prishtina and Mitrovitza, in addition to the evaluation of the patients we made several journeys, distributing hospital material, of which the local hospitals were almost entirely destitute; the men were lying on the floor on straw like cattle, and the mortality from pneumonia was terrible. There were two reasons for this: in the first place, the enemy had taken away or destroyed all hospital and other stores; and in the second, transport into Central Serbia had broken-down completely, the bridges, even the smallest, having been destroyed. There was an epidemic of Spanish influenza among the M.T. companies,[3] and owing to the unexpectedly rapid advance and the breaking of the weather, a tremendous strain was put on the motor

---

3. The British Tommies we read of later in the S.W.H. at Vranja were drawn largely from the M.T. companies.

transport systems, and there were of course no railways at all. We gained a little insight into what war prices could be when we were told that coffee, when obtainable, was 250 *francs* a kilo, and a reel of cotton had cost 23s.

Farther north towards Belgrade things were a little better, though food and hospital requisites were terribly scarce. Everywhere we were received with the most touching cordiality and hospitality; in many of the towns we passed through they had never seen an Englishwoman before, much less a woman chauffeur—in fact, they had to invent a new feminine form of the word 'chauffeur' to meet the emergency.

At Uzice we found that the mountain passes into Bosnia had become impracticable—ten men and four oxen failed to get a Ford van through—so we turned back, and, passing through Mladanovatz, with its broken fountain, reached Belgrade on 18th December.

While we were in Belgrade we and the Yellak Unit were inspected by the prince regent, and received decorations from him. The gold medal received by the drivers is a valuable decoration not often given. We were now under orders to rejoin our own hospital at Sarajevo, and as there is no bridge over the Danube we had to ask for a barge from Admiral Troubridge and drive the cars on to it. This was a rather dangerous proceeding—the front wheels of one car shot over the edge of the barge, and we nearly lost car and driver in the Save. Then we drove the cars on to railway trucks, and after a sleepless but amusing night in the waiting-room we left Semlin on Christmas Day at about 8 a.m., and finished our journey by rail. We had secured a Christmas turkey in Belgrade, and he created some consternation by disappearing at Semlin; a vigorous search, however, discovered him in an empty petrol can.

When we reached Sarajevo we found ourselves in civilisation again, and at the end of the most interesting part of our work, but we never succeeded in reaching the end of the kindness of our Serbian and Jugo-Slav friends: no words could exaggerate the cordiality and hospitality with which we were treated by the Serbian officers or by our civilian friends in Cacak, Sarajevo, or Zagreb. It made one feel deeply grateful to have had an opportunity of doing anything, however small, to bring about the enfranchisement of so fine a people.

It has been wonderful to hear on all sides in Belgrade of the magnificent work done by Miss Dillon's and Miss Robinson's transports. Every soldier and officer I met spoke most enthusiastically of our women drivers, and of their heroism during the last advance. Especially admired was their *sang-froid* when something went wrong with their ambulances, and shells and aeroplanes were about.[4]

---

4. From a private letter to the (original) editor.

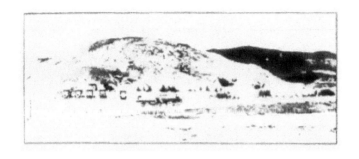

A GROUP OF TENTS AT OSTROVO

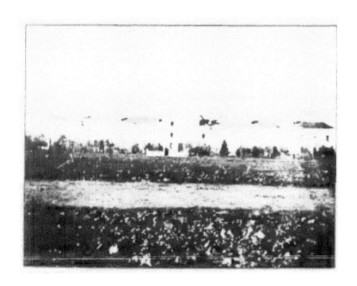

VRANJA

CHAPTER 4

Vranja

We have seen how the round of work the Scottish Women were proud to do for Serbia was completed by their entry into Belgrade with the triumphant army. But though the circle was completed, the work by no means came to an end when the Transport Column was demobilised. If we are still to follow the Scottish Women in their last venture, we must retrace our steps from Belgrade back past the familiar-sounding names in the north till we reach the town of Vranja in the centre of Serbia. Here we shall find in November 1918 the Unit from Ostrovo, now under Dr. Emslie, who had moved from their beautiful camp by the lake there, to take over from the Serbs the hospital at Vranja.

This was a huge building with a long frontage and wings jutting out to the back at each end. It was formerly a barracks, and required much attention before it could properly fulfil the new requirements. As the hospital was the only one within a radius of fifty miles, it was full to overflowing with patients; but much had to be done in the way of cleaning and making provision for lighting and for hot water—no easy task in the case of such a large building.

In the delightful letter which follows, written by Mrs. Green, administrator to the unit, we get a detailed account of the move from Ostrovo to Vranja, and of the work the unit had to do on their immediate arrival.

Vranja, Serbia, 4th November.
I know you will be wondering where we are and what we are doing. As you know, the advance on the Balkan front came very suddenly, and things happened before one could think or realise what was happening. About a month ago we had orders

from our Director of Medical Service to evacuate all patients, and prepare to go to Serbia at once, as our help was urgently needed. Every one helped with a right good will, Matron and Miss Barker doing colossal work. Dr. Emslie and I started for Serbia to see where our hospital was to be. Miss West drove us nearly all the way, and we took a Serb driver with us also as we were anxious to do the trip in as short a time as possible, and arranged that Miss West and the Serb should relieve one another.

The first day we got as far as Skoplje, and that, in spite of having to pass many Bulgarian *dursins* leaving Serbia. They looked tolerably well cared for, and not as if they had been starved or neglected in any way. Officers and men saluted us as we passed. We arrived at Skoplje about 8 o'clock at night, and got a room in the Hospital where Colonel Vladosavlovitch was staying. He was delighted to find that we were moving so quickly, and said that the need for us was very terrible. Next day we started early and arrived at Vranja about 6 o'clock.

The hospital is an enormous building, and was originally used as a barracks. Doctors and students were working night and day, and patients were pouring in all the time. The doctors attached to the ambulance wanted us to take charge at once, but of course we could not. They were anxious to get on behind the army, where the need was even greater.

Next day we returned to Skoplje, where we spent the night, and again saw Vladosavlovitch, who told us that he could not help us in any way about transport, as all the Serbian convoys had gone on to Nish; however, he begged us to try to help the Serbs, as there were no doctors or nurses available to do anything. Dr. Emslie reassured him by telling him that we had already arranged for the removal of our personnel and for part of our equipment at least—the most necessary things to start our work with. I may tell you that the prospects were appalling, hundreds of patients wanting help of every kind, and practically no food in the country—coffee, £4 a kilo; tea, £4, 10s.; sugar, 35 *drs.*, or about £1, 10s. a kilo, and everything in proportion, and very little to be got even at those prices so that the day after we arrived at Ostrovo I hurried down to Salonika to collect all the food, drugs, and equipment that I could manage to get.

General Fortescue was very good, and gave me permission to

buy what I wanted from the British Ordnance. The Red Cross people also were very good, and gave me 100 sheets, 100 pillow-slips, 100 prs. socks, 100 prs. pyjamas. 6 sacks flour, 100 lbs. sugar, 2 boxes of milk, 1 case coffee, and a few other things. We got all the equipment packed on to the railway wagons, and Dr. Blake and three of the orderlies went with it to Monastir.

Before I go further, I must tell you how absolutely overjoyed we were to find that our long-looked-for Selden lorry had arrived in Salonika in time to help us to bring our sisters here. Our old Selden and the G.M.C. lorry took all our stuff to the railway station, so that we did not need any outside help at all. The Kelly Springfield lorry made many journeys to the station, but finally broke its axle and had lo be sent to Salonika to be repaired, so that the new Selden got a wonderful reception when we got back to Ostrovo with it. We were a most imposing-looking convoy when we started with 2 touring-cars, small Ford van, 3 ambulances, 2 Seldens, and the G.M.C. lorry. There were so many sisters in each, with the bare necessaries of life in their haversacks, and food enough for a five days' journey. Each car carried a small Serbian flag which we had made, and the leading car had a small Union Jack.

All our sisters were in splendid spirits at the prospect of really good work, and all were in excellent health; and I felt very thankful, as Spanish influenza was very bad here, and I was anxious that they should all keep fit. In Monastir I met a man who had trekked through Albania with us, and we had shared our food with him, so he was anxious to help us. He was running a Y.M.C.A. canteen, and he gave us a place behind his tents for our wagons to stand for the night. His men made tea for the whole formidable party, and gave us tables and benches so that we could have our supper in comfort. Each member of our unit was allowed to carry a small haversack containing necessaries, also a camp bed, ground sheet, pillow, and two blankets, so that we were able to be quite comfortable.

We were lucky enough to have lovely moonlight for our journey, and it was rather a wonderful sight to see our rows of little beds with the sisters sleeping placidly, while a few yards away guns, ammunition, and soldiers of many nationalities passed along in a steady stream. We were up bright and early, and soon ready. As our car was leading and doing so well. Dr. Emslie suggested that we should hurry on and try to get some place for the Unit to sleep in al Veles. In all the villages through which we passed we found Serbian flags flying, and everyone looking relieved and expectant, as of course the Serbs were hurrying back as fast as ever they could to their homes.

We arrived in Veles about 8 o'clock, and were lucky enough to find two of the 'Elsie Inglis' Unit, who took us to the house where they had got rooms for the night. Our party did not turn up, but spent the night at the top of the Babuna Pass, where the Serbs once fought so valiantly, and they did not arrive until about 2 o'clock next day. As the Selden had not put in an appearance, we decided to spend the night in Veles, and the Serbian Prefect gave us the village school to sleep in. I had to forage round and get food for my unit, and fortunately I was able to get enough for them all, though food was certainly very scarce and a terrible price.

Next day we started early, after I had raided the British canteen and collected as much food as possible for the remainder of the journey. The day was fine and sunny, and some of the scenery through which we passed was very wonderful. Up and down over those beautiful mountains we went, passing and repassing endless streams of traffic going and coming over hills and passes, until we came to a small village where we had lunch. This consisted of tongue—which we had got from the British canteen—and bread, as well as tomatoes, cheese, and pears, which I bought in the village, so that we had quite a banquet in the main street with all the inhabitants looking on. That night we got to Skoplje about dusk, and went to Lady Paget's old hospital, where we found some of the Serbian Relief people busy getting the place into order.

They were very kind and helped us to get hot water for tea, and we spent quite a comfortable night there. After supper we went to see Dr. Chesney and her people, who had just arrived to work there; their hospital was quite full, and everyone was very busy. Lots of our old patients greeted us in Skoplje. We were glad to find that the town had not been very much destroyed, but most of the railway bridges and telegraph and telephone systems were blown up, and there was useless and wanton waste everywhere.

We arrived in Vranja about 8 o'clock, and felt our spirits a little damped, as the night was very cold and it was raining; hard, and no preparations had been made for us; however, we soon got beds put up in one of the wards, and after rather a scanty supper we went to bed. In the morning we found the ground white with snow, and the cold intense. The Serbian ambulance left the hospital about 6 o'clock in the morning, and we all set to work to do what we could to get some of the wards cleaned up.

Patients had simply poured into Vranja during the advance, and at times there were 1500 patients stowed away in all sorts of odd corners, but by the time we arrived there were only about 400. Four Serbian doctors and a few medical students had worked heroically, and treated not only the wounded and sick in hospital, but all the people in the town who were suffering from Spanish influenza. They had done splendid work, but. as you can imagine, there was no time for cleaning or keeping sanitary arrangements in any kind of order, so that our tasks at first seemed almost too enormous.

Miss Barker has been a perfect tower of strength, and has tackled the most appalling and disgusting difficulties with splendid courage and cheeriness. I can never say enough for the way every one has buckled to and worked, and it has been work under the very greatest possible difficulties, as we did not possess a single brush, duster, pail, nor a single piece of soap, and yet the wards got cleaned with brushes made from branches cut from the trees round the hospital. They have performed wonders in one short week, but, as you can imagine, there is a great deal still to be done.

This is an enormous building, originally used as a barracks, and there are many outhouses of all sorts, a good garage with concrete floor, excellent places for storing all our things. We are terribly badly needed, as there is no doctor in the place, and such an amount of illness. In one of the wards we found several English Tommies suffering very much from influenza: one especially, a boy H———, was very ill and died next morning. We were glad to be here and see that he was decently buried. We made a wreath and cross of lovely flowers, and as many nurses as could get away went to his funeral. His comrades carried him to the cemetery, and Dr. Emslie read a short burial service at the grave.

We did feel so sad that we had not been able to come a day or two sooner; however, the doctor and sisters have done wonders for the other boys, and they are improving wonderfully. We have eleven of them in at present, and all sorts of people come craving to be admitted, so that I think it would be difficult to find a more cosmopolitan hospital anywhere.

I don't suppose the censor would like me to tell you too much about the awful condition of things here. The people say the Germans took all the food and useful material of every kind out of the country before they left, so that the deprivation has been terrible: but we are going to do all that we can for the poor suffering people here, and I can assure you that the efforts of the S.W. H are much appreciated by everyone—the Serbs, French, and British. If it is possible, we want all the warm clothing we can get—shirts, pyjamas, socks, mufflers, bedding, blankets; everything is needed badly; men, women, and children are nearly naked. The roads, of course, will be very difficult during the winter, but we are hoping that the railway from Salonika will soon be repaired, and that we can get things brought up more easily.

Forgive a hurried, incoherent, rambling, letter, but Miss S——, one of Miss Dillon's girls, has just come in from Nish *en route* for England, and I want to sent this by her in the morning, so that you will know what we are doing.

"I have sat up nearly all night to write it, and I have had a very strenuous day. We are working hard and the suffering and sadness all round one are simply terrible. A poor Serbian officer was brought in unconscious two nights ago. Today he insisted upon getting up and going on to Skoplje. He was most unfit to go out, and Dr. Emslie and I did our best to persuade him to remain for a night or two longer. Then he told us his pitiful tale, how he had gone up into Serbia with his heart full of joy and hope that, after three years of separation, he was to see his wife and little children again in the home he loved. But he had found it burnt to the ground and a new coffee-house arranged in the ruins, and his wife and little children hanged by the Bulgars.

He said he was only one of many officers who had the same experience. 'Most of them shot themselves or went mad, but I have come on to find my regiment, as my men were left behind at Skoplje and may not be able to get rations until I return.

When I have made arrangements for them I will take something to make me sleep and sleep! I am not ill at all with any ordinary curable illness, but just my heart is broken, and I don't want to live.' I took him to the mess-room and gave him Serbian coffee, and got him to eat a little, and it seemed to comfort him to talk, but he insisted on leaving the hospital and going off to Skoplje. I fear there is terrible suffering and sorrow in store for many of the poor Serbs, and the end of the war will only mean the beginning of fresh sorrows for many of them.

On the other hand, there will be some happy meetings. I brought letters and a parcel from a doctor in Vodena to his wife and children who live here, and it was delightful to see their joy. His two children threw their arms round me and begged me to take them to daddy. His wife was very quiet, and unable to realise that her husband was really alive, but his old mother's joy was too wonderful. He was her only son, and she had mourned for him for three years, as they told her that he was dead! And so the time goes on—interesting things happening all the while, and the days never long enough for all that has got to be done. When I feel extra tired I go into the English Tommies' ward, and it revives me to see them looking so comfortable and so appreciative.

Dr. Emslie, C.M.O. of the unit at Vranja, had worked with the S.W.H. in the Girton and Newnham Unit, under Dr. Louise M'Ilroy, since 1915. She has done wonders at Vranja. It is no easy task to take over a hospital full of patients, which has been carried on without a sufficient staff of doctors, with no nurses and no proper organisation, and to convert it into an orderly and efficient institution. It was this task which faced Dr. Emslie at Vranja, and which she performed with marked courage and success. In the quotations from her letters which follow, the story of Vranja is continued.

From other sources we learn of the candle-lit corridors and wards in the first weeks before electric light was installed, and of the ward full for many a day of British Tommies—"our own Boys," as Dr. Inglis called them.

Vranja, 9th November 1918.
It will be a fortnight tomorrow evening since we arrived at Vranja, and it seems years already. All of us arrived together, as we kept a convoy the whole way. We took five days to do the

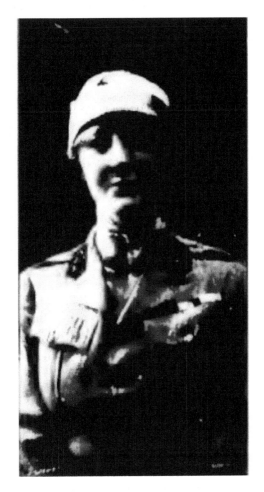

Dr. Isabel Emslie

trek. Mrs. Green managed the food part so well that we always had enough to eat. I shall try to write you, later on, all about that journey, with its interests and its pathos, its dangers and difficulties.

I felt very much the responsibility of bringing all the staff here, and the great difficulty of getting our material up however, I saw that here in Vranja was the place for work. I never have seen work like it, and so I determined by any means to get the unit up there.

I had them all together at Ostrovo, told them about the difficulties and dangers, and gave them the chance of going home. They decided to come on, and here we are at Vranja, and *nearly all our material*, which has to come the whole way from Monastir to Vranja in lorries.

I cannot say how much we owe to the heads of the French and British Transports, who have put us before everybody else, including themselves, in giving us transport. They have not any hospitals yet of their own—only two small detention-tent hospitals for the British, and these fifty and a hundred miles from here. The British have asked us to take the Tommies, which we are very glad to do—and they much appreciate being with us. We have all nationalities—French, English, Serb, Roumanian, Bulgar, Austrian, and German, officers and men—and Colonel Vladosavlovitch has told us to receive any of the Allies.

When we arrived here, we found an absolutely filthy building with 450 very ill patients in it—each case almost a problem in itself. The medical cases nearly all were broncho-pneumonia or pneumonia, pleurisy and empyaemia—most of them very serious; and the surgical cases were appalling—many needing operation, and all the dressings were just as they had been first put on.

We had an out-patient department running on until 7 p.m. in the evening—chiefly women and children from the village, where the conditions are just awful at present. They have had no doctors all this time, and still have none, and are in very bad condition from poor feeding. We have had already to do a great many immediate operations on children who have been wounded by bombs and still are being wounded by the shells exploding. The injuries are terrible, and we have had several poor little hands to amputate, and often they have terrible ab-

338

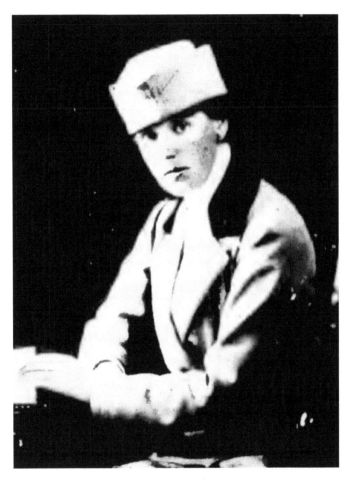

DR. LOUISE M'ILROY

dominal wounds. These children we have got to take in, but all other civilians we are keeping out in the meantime, as we have far too many soldiers as it is. Perhaps later on we may be able to take in and operate on some of the most imperative civilian cases.

We have had to do a few urgent cases in the village, and Dr. McKenzie and I try each to go there for an hour a day; it is really our recreation, even though one is working the whole time in the village—it is a change. It is heart-breaking not to be able to look after everyone and receive all who want to come to hospital, but unfortunately the day is only twenty-four hours long and our hospital has not elastic sides.

The hospital will actually hold 300 beds comfortably when we are settled, as one wing I have shut off for a nurses' home, and part of the other for an outpatients' department. If we are still here in summer, however, I shall put the whole nursing staff in tents.

I have wired you for ten nurses and one doctor, preferably with some laboratory experience, so that she could run the laboratory, typhoid, dysentery, and malaria work especially.

Dr. Blake and Dr. McKenzie seem to be enjoying the work immensely, and are at it from morning till night, and often during the night. We are all awfully happy together, and everybody seems to be enjoying every minute of the work.

Vranja, 8th December 1918

We are still just as busy as we were when we first arrived, and I think we are likely to be so all the winter, as there seems to be no probability of other hospitals coming to Vranja. Nish and Skoplje are the nearest and even there they are dreadfully overworked. We are trying to keep our numbers down in hospital, but what can one do when dying people come and sit on one's doorstep? We always said the greatest work would be done when the Serbs arrived back in Serbia but conditions are even worse than we thought they would be.

We are gradually getting the place quite smart and very soon it will be free of smells. The nurses' home wing is absolutely clean, has a bathing-room, and a plentiful supply of hot water. It is quite shut off from the rest of the hospital, and is entered by a separate side door.

The mess-room is in a separate building just close beside the hospital and in the grounds, and there also is the kitchen, the washing-up room, and a huge room which used to be full of Bulgars in the last stage all sorts of disease. Now I shall have it cleaned and kept for a recreation-room, and also for the patients who are able to be up for meals. At present, we have practically none fit to be up, for as soon as they are able to get out of bed they have to be sent off all the way up to Nish, or down to Skoplje.

Vranja, 12th January 1919.

The work increases daily, instead of showing any signs of decreasing. I am now unable even to get the number of patients below 350, however hard I try, and it is generally about 367. We still are able to take in only the very worst cases, and accidents and operations, and have to turn away nearly all the Bulgars, unless very ill. The latter are in a dreadful state—hardly any food or clothes, sometimes they are two or three days without food. One morning we had three brought in, one of whom was dead; another sat down on the doorstep and died, and the third died on the stretcher on his way to the ward. This may just give you a faint idea of conditions. It is not the authorities' fault, for the roads are so bad and it is so difficult to get food up, and the way to our hospital so long, that the men cannot stand the walk.

We are the only doctors in Vranja, or for that matter within a radius of fifty mile? At the *Komanda Mesta* (Commandant de la Place) I still do the *Komicia* (Medical Board) for the recruits, and for the soldiers leaving the army. There is no military doctor to do this.

We have been here now ten weeks and six days, and are very comfortable. We have got electric light up in all the wards, theatre, and administrative part, and our engine is running very well. The question of wood for heating and cooking is a little easier now, and life is not quite so difficult.

We feel almost civilised with the train only forty miles away.

Vranja, 15th February 1919.

. . . I have expected since our first day here to have cases of typhus, but all went well till this spell of cold weather came. For the past fortnight we have had deep snow, and sunless, miserable weather, and with it came the typhus. I believe they have the same outbreaks in Nish and Skoplje, and in Bulgaria, but it is difficult to hear any definite news. They have also some small-pox. I don't think this will be a big epidemic, and we are taking every possible care, and have reminded the town authorities about precautions. The people have no one to help or advise them, so we have to do the best we can for them.

While the typhus is on, I have stopped the Bulgar patients coming to the hospital. We were getting crowded out with them, and if we had a two-thousand-bed hospital we should not have enough beds. Poor wretches most of them are hardly like men at all. A number have frozen feet now, and all are wasted, and many demented. We still sometimes have as many as half a dozen brought in on willow stretchers moribund, having fallen out on the way to hospital. It is the most ghastly sight.

I am afraid these poor Bulgars are having a dreadful time in their camps, but I considered, all round, it was best not to risk overcrowding while this epidemic lasts.

I have also stopped all but the most urgent off patient dressings till the typhus blows over. I hope it may soon finish, as the town, the out-patients, and the Bulgars are suffering while it lasts.

9th April 1919.

Typhus still continues. We have over 100 cases in hospital, and the epidemic is not abating as quickly as I thought it would.

The question of food gives us no trouble now. Rations are coming in regularly, and they are good, patients' and staff ration money is coming in daily. There is a sufficiency of wood and everything else. All these things are largely due to the train service which now runs direct from Salonika to Vranja, and up to Nish, but no nearer Belgrade than that.

I told you we had taken over a German laundry when we came first, 'complete with every modern convenience.' We have now fifteen women working in it and six scrubbers in the hospital. The authorities have agreed to pay all these people for us, so we are getting much more economical.

The hospital begins to look smarter, and the grounds are beginning to look lovely. Our garden is simply blooming with apple, pear, plum, and peach, and the lilacs are going to burst in a day or two. There are very many in the garden. With the help of a

British sergeant and some old Serbs and Bulgars a very successful tennis court has been made, and has been in use for the past rive days. It is mud and sand, and plays well. The Red Cross gave us the posts and net and balls.

Hockey continues three times a week, and in the meantime all are keeping fit.

The *prefect* of Vranja has given us a beautiful little villa at Vranski Banja, and there we shall send any 'tired' or convalescent staff. It is an empty house, very new and clean, and was used before the war as the doctor's residence in connection with the hot springs. Vranski Banja is a Serbian 'Baden-Baden,' and was before the war a very fashionable place; certainly the houses are much better built than anything I have so far seen in Serbia, but no 'fashionables' have yet arrived, I am glad to say.

Our villa has two balconies—one along the side and one round the front door. It stands right up on the hill and has a gorgeous view and a nice garden. I think we are very lucky to have it given to us, and I am sure it will be most useful. It is just seven miles from the hospital, so it will be easy to reach.

I have not told you of our one Serbian probationer. We hope shortly to have more, as she is proving such a success. She is Olga Achinovitch. We have dressed her in blue-and-white striped overall, with white collar and cuffs, and small Quaker cap, turned back with white. She comes regularly and works very hard.

Bishop Price and Colonel Findlay (*padre*) have been staying with us for two days on a mission to the troops. The bishop left for Nish today and returns in a few days to conduct service in our hall on Sunday, for ourselves and the British M.T. men. Our hut makes a fine church, and in it three days ago there was solemnised a wedding—that of a British M.T. corporal and a charming Serbian girl. She looked so sweet in white, with veil and orange blossom. Mr. Green and I thought we ought to make some effort to have it all very nice—not only because we knew the couple, but because of the alliance of the nations, as the whole countryside knew of the wedding. It was absolutely English, except that a Serbian priest and crowds of Serbian people were present.

Twenty of us were in the choir. We wore white overalls and white veils, and carried bunches of lilac. About the same number of M. T. men were in the choir also. We had forms on each side arranged like choir stalls, and an aisle formed by sisters, holding long garlands and lilac. We all thought it was the prettiest wedding we had ever seen, and it was just arranged the evening before. The girls are so good the way they rise to things when they are often dead tired. They all looked very nice at the wedding, and so bright and happy, and there was no evidence of hurry, though everyone had to tear back to the wards again just as soon as the ceremony was finished.

Mrs. Green had a very busy time in Salonika and a very successful one. The Red Cross, through Colonel Fitzpatrick, have been even more generous than ever before, and have given us seven or more truck loads—large size—of Red Cross Store, including clothing, food stuffs, and hospital equipment. Colonel Fitzpatrick hopes to come and see us in about a month's time, on his way to Belgrade.

Vranja, 28th May 1919.

Dear Mrs. Russell.—Many thanks for your letter of the 29th April, and also for the medals which arrived by Sister Aitken. We are all charmed with them. I think they are most beautifully designed and finished. The workmanship is so fine, and each little detail—the barette even—is so perfect. I have heard several of the sisters say, 'I'd much rather wear this than any other medal I could get.' We are wearing it on the right side, more as a hospital badge.

Our coming and going members are being put up at the American Red Cross in Salonika now, with which Society we are on the most friendly terms. The M.T.O. advises the American Red Cross at once of their arrival, and it is all very simple and comfortable. We give them hospitality here when they pass, and they give us a great deal of material one way and another.

The Serbian Relief Fund, too, are giving Mrs. Green a quantity of clothing for distribution. We are on very good terms with this Society too. They are most accommodating in putting up our members passing through Skoplje, and we are hardly ever without some of their people passing through or coming for a few days' holiday.

The villa at Vranski Banje is in full swing. It looks more charming than ever. It is well built, and is certainly quite the most modern-looking house I have seen in Vranja. It has three bedrooms and one sitting-room, all done up most tastefully by Miss Munn, a very good kitchen, and a new garden and two large verandahs. There is also room for the man and his wife who live out there always. She cooks and cleans, and he attends to the outside arrangements and, as he is by trade a bootmaker, mend shoes for the hospital.

Then I have a room for a dispensary there with doors of its own and a separate entrance to the house. The people come from the surrounding villages for dressings, medicines, and to have their eyes and ears looked after. At present I have the two American nurses lent by the American Red Cross out there, and they are working the dispensary. They get on so well with all our girls, and it is so nice to have an inter-Ally feeling about it. I am getting things from the Americans, too, to stock this dispensary. They are all very keen about it.

I am running a lorry out there three times a week with supplies, and it should carry about six members with it each time. They love going to out little home, and the whole place is just a fairyland of flowers.

We never get below our three hundred and forty patients, and are not even yet admitting all; but now we are able to take in cervical adenitis and more chronic cases for operation, and hope soon to have a fifteen-bedded ward instead of our present six-bedded room for women. (It really has ten in it.) We hope soon also to have a children's ward. Typhus has practically ceased now, and all the staff at present are absolutely fit. We have therefore taken the opportunity of doing up the sisters' sick-room. It is done in natural holland (from the Red Cross) and that beautiful cretonne you sent us. It is in shades of blue, purple, and rose and everything is arranged to match—a little cretonne settee, cushions, and electric light shade, etc. We are doing the officers' ward up in practically the same style.

I told you in my last letter of the tuberculosis patients that Prince Alexander's Hospital wished us to take. We are able now to receive them, so seventeen of them are coming quite soon. We are putting a tent up for the ones that are pretty well, and the others will go into a ward and will stay out in the verandahs all day and perhaps, later on, at night.

We have had steady rain for six weeks now, except for perhaps two or three hours' sunshine in the afternoon. In spite of this the garden is getting on, the seeds are all coming up and soon will be ready for transplanting, and the rose trees are just covered with buds.

We have great help in the outside work by two English soldiers, Ecklorff and Doran, left behind with us by their companies. We hope to get permission to keep them till they are demobilised. They work a squad of Bulgars. It is charming to see how these men get on with an Englishman.

We have still a few British Tommies in hospital. When they are well they will be sent to Salonika to report for home.

It was rather touching how when the English Companies left here several of the Tommies came to me and asked if they could stay to 'protect' us, as they couldn't bear the thought of leaving us all alone in Vranja. . . .

The work of this hospital in Vranja—the last of the Scottish Women's Hospitals to be closed—recalls in many respects the labours of the other units, and, combining memories of them all, leads us towards the close of the history.

As we read of the cleaning, that had to be done on their arrival, and of the staff finding their way about the enormous building by the dim light of candles, we are reminded of the first fortnight in the Abbey of Royaumont.

The typhus epidemic fought so bravely carries us back in memory to Kraguievatz, where the Scottish Women's connection with Serbia began.

And the British Tommies, as they streamed into the hospital with their oft-repeated "Ah Sister if the Scottish Women had been here sooner none of us would have died!" remind us of the original idea of the founders of the S.W.H. when their first unit magnificently equipped, and with a C.M.O. of Miss Iven's calibre, was offered to the British War Office. Red tape blocked the way to its acceptance. But with the quiet force which comes from patience, and from the determination to serve always where they were most needed, the Scottish Women attained in, the end their primary object, having previous to its fulfilment served in a wider field and on more extensive battle fronts than even their fearless founder had dreamed of in 1914.

From a British Mother:

To Dr. Emslie, c/o Scottish Women's Hospital,
    Vranja, Serbia

Dear Dr. Emslie,—I cannot refrain from writing you a short note, to say how grateful and pleased I an to hear of the very great kindness and tender care which yourself and your staff of the above hospital have shown towards my son and the other boys under your charge. I also realise that yourself and your staff are working under difficulties very great indeed, which I can hardly believe to be true. I have indeed been comforted by the knowledge that all was done for the best, and I am sure that the other mothers of this country who have also got sons on active service in your area will also appreciate what has been done for them.

Accept, dear friend, my deepest thanks, which is all I can offer.—Yours faithfully,

(Sgd.)   Mrs. M——.

Note—The hospital at Vranja was closed in October 1918, Dr. Emslie taking up the work of C.M.O. in the Elsie Inglis Memorial Hospital.

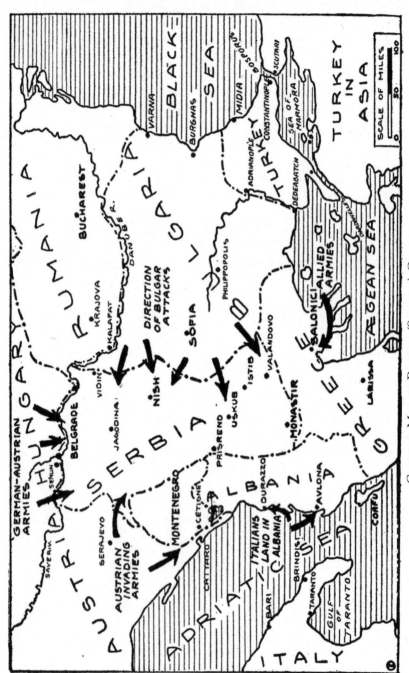

General Map of Balkan (Serbian) Operations.

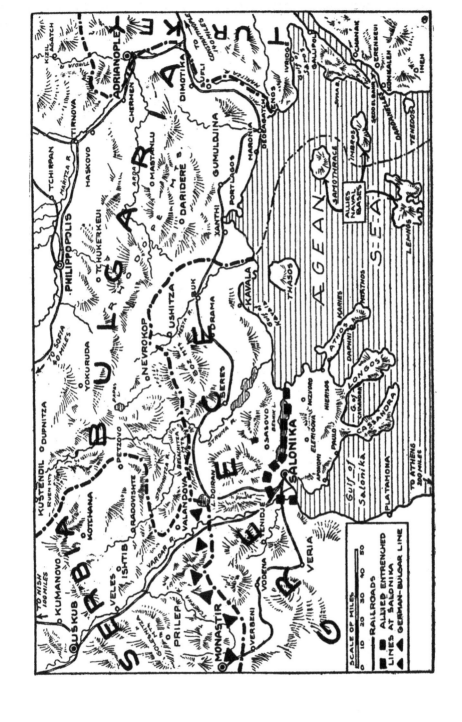

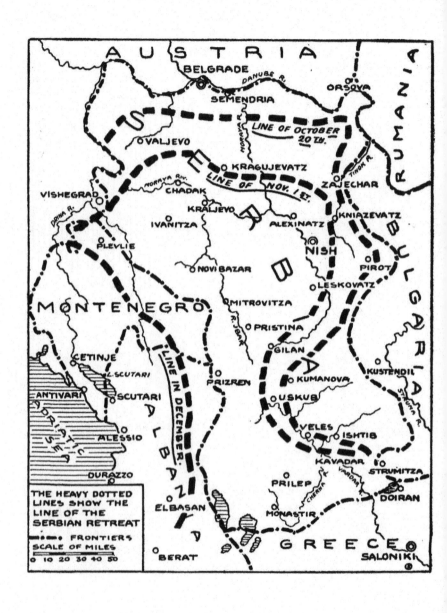

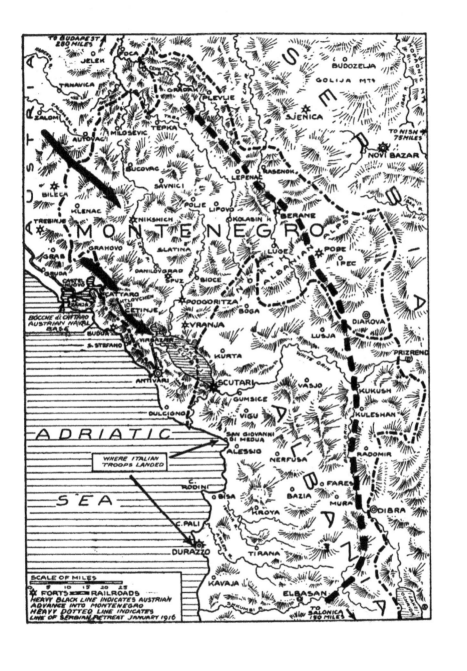

LEONAUR

ALSO FROM LEONAUR
AVAILABLE IN SOFTCOVER OR HARDCOVER WITH DUST JACKET

A DIARY FROM DIXIE by Mary Boykin Chesnut—A Lady's Account of the Confederacy During the American Civil War

FOLLOWING THE DRUM by Teresa Griffin Vielé—A U. S. Infantry Officer's Wife on the Texas frontier in the Early 1850's

FOLLOWING THE GUIDON by Elizabeth B. Custer—The Experiences of General Custer's Wife with the U. S. 7th Cavalry.

LADIES OF LUCKNOW by G. Harris & Adelaide Case—The Experiences of Two British Women During the Indian Mutiny 1857. A Lady's Diary of the Siege of Lucknow by G. Harris, Day by Day at Lucknow by Adelaide Case

MARIE-LOUISE AND THE INVASION OF 1814 by Imbert de Saint-Amand—The Empress and the Fall of the First Empire

SAPPER DOROTHY by Dorothy Lawrence—The only English Woman Soldier in the Royal Engineers 51st Division, 79th Tunnelling Co. during the First World War

ARMY LETTERS FROM AN OFFICER'S WIFE 1871-1888 by Frances M. A. Roe—Experiences On the Western Frontier With the United States Army

NAPOLEON'S LETTERS TO JOSEPHINE by Henry Foljambe Hall—Correspondence of War, Politics, Family and Love 1796-1814

MEMOIRS OF SARAH DUCHESS OF MARLBOROUGH, AND OF THE COURT OF QUEEN ANNE VOLUME 1 by A. T. Thomson

MEMOIRS OF SARAH DUCHESS OF MARLBOROUGH, AND OF THE COURT OF QUEEN ANNE VOLUME 2 by A. T. Thomson

MARY PORTER GAMEWELL AND THE SIEGE OF PEKING by A. H. Tuttle—An American Lady's Experiences of the Boxer Uprising, China 1900

VANISHING ARIZONA by Martha Summerhayes—A young wife of an officer of the U.S. 8th Infantry in Apacheria during the 1870's

THE RIFLEMAN'S WIFE by Mrs. Fitz Maurice—*The Experiences of an Officer's Wife and Chronicles of the Old 95th During the Napoleonic Wars*

THE OATMAN GIRLS by Royal B. Stratton—The Capture & Captivity of Two Young American Women in the 1850's by the Apache Indians

LEONAUR

ALSO FROM LEONAUR

AVAILABLE IN SOFTCOVER OR HARDCOVER WITH DUST JACKET

THE WOMAN IN BATTLE *by Loreta Janeta Velazquez*—Soldier, Spy and Secret Service Agent for the Confederacy During the American Civil War.

BOOTS AND SADDLES *by Elizabeth B. Custer*—The experiences of General Custer's Wife on the Western Plains.

FANNIE BEERS' CIVIL WAR *by Fannie A. Beers*—A Confederate Lady's Experiences of Nursing During the Campaigns & Battles of the American Civil War.

LADY SALE'S AFGHANISTAN *by Florentia Sale*—An Indomitable Victorian Lady's Account of the Retreat from Kabul During the First Afghan War.

THE TWO WARS OF MRS DUBERLY *by Frances Isabella Duberly*—An Intrepid Victorian Lady's Experience of the Crimea and Indian Mutiny.

THE REBELLIOUS DUCHESS *by Paul F. S. Dermoncourt*—The Adventures of the Duchess of Berri and Her Attempt to Overthrow French Monarchy.

LADIES OF WATERLOO *by Charlotte A. Eaton, Magdalene de Lancey & Juana Smith*—The Experiences of Three Women During the Campaign of 1815: Waterloo Days by Charlotte A. Eaton, A Week at Waterloo by Magdalene de Lancey & Juana's Story by Juana Smith.

NURSE AND SPY IN THE UNION ARMY *by Sarah Emma Evelyn Edmonds*—During the American Civil War

WIFE NO. 19 *by Ann Eliza Young*—The Life & Ordeals of a Mormon Woman During the 19th Century

DIARY OF A NURSE IN SOUTH AFRICA *by Alice Bron*—With the Dutch-Belgian Red Cross During the Boer War

MARIE ANTOINETTE AND THE DOWNFALL OF ROYALTY *by Imbert de Saint-Amand*—The Queen of France and the French Revolution

THE MEMSAHIB & THE MUTINY *by R. M. Coopland*—An English lady's ordeals in Gwalior and Agra duringthe Indian Mutiny 1857

MY CAPTIVITY AMONG THE SIOUX INDIANS *by Fanny Kelly*—The ordeal of a pioneer woman crossing the Western Plains in 1864

WITH MAXIMILIAN IN MEXICO *by Sara Yorke Stevenson*—A Lady's experience of the French Adventure

LEONAUR

ALSO FROM LEONAUR
AVAILABLE IN SOFTCOVER OR HARDCOVER WITH DUST JACKET